# ETHICS FOR COUNSELORS

**Silvia L. Mazzula, PhD,** has over a decade of experience in curriculum development, including developing and teaching train-the-trainer programs for mental health providers. In her role as a professor, Dr. Mazzula teaches courses on forensic mental health counseling, group treatment, and multicultural psychology. She also specializes in culturally competent treatment of diverse clients. Dr. Mazzula graduated from The College of New Jersey with an MA in counseling and human services (CACREP accredited) and from Columbia University with a PhD in counseling psychology (APA accredited).

**Pamela LiVecchi, PsyD,** has spent the last decade creating and providing trainings focused on effective self-care and ethical behavior. In her role as a therapist, Dr. LiVecchi has worked with clients in a variety of settings, providing individual and group psychotherapy, as well as psychological evaluations. She also specializes in teaching students who work within the substance abuse and forensic fields. Dr. LiVecchi graduated from Argosy University–Northern Virginia with a PsyD in clinical psychology (APA accredited).

# ETHICS FOR COUNSELORS
## Integrating Counseling and Psychology Standards

*Silvia L. Mazzula, PhD*
*Pamela LiVecchi, PsyD*

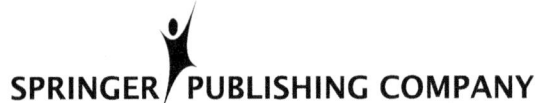

Copyright © 2018 Springer Publishing Company, LLC

All rights reserved.

No part of this publication may be reproduced, stored in a retrieval system, or transmitted in any form or by any means, electronic, mechanical, photocopying, recording, or otherwise, without the prior permission of Springer Publishing Company, LLC, or authorization through payment of the appropriate fees to the Copyright Clearance Center, Inc., 222 Rosewood Drive, Danvers, MA 01923, 978-750-8400, fax 978-646-8600, info@copyright.com or on the Web at www.copyright.com.

Springer Publishing Company, LLC
11 West 42nd Street
New York, NY 10036
www.springerpub.com

*Acquisitions Editor*: Sheri W. Sussman
*Compositor*: S4Carlisle Publishing Services

*ISBN*: 9780826181862
*ebook ISBN*: 9780826181817

*Instructors' Materials: Qualified instructors may request supplements by emailing textbook@springerpub.com:*
*Instructors' Manual ISBN:* 9780826181848
*Instructors' PowerPoints ISBN:* 9780826181855

17 18 19 20 21 / 5 4 3 2 1

The author and the publisher of this Work have made every effort to use sources believed to be reliable to provide information that is accurate and compatible with the standards generally accepted at the time of publication. The author and publisher shall not be liable for any special, consequential, or exemplary damages resulting, in whole or in part, from the readers' use of, or reliance on, the information contained in this book. The publisher has no responsibility for the persistence or accuracy of URLs for external or third-party Internet websites referred to in this publication and does not guarantee that any content on such websites is, or will remain, accurate or appropriate.

**Library of Congress Cataloging-in-Publication Data**

Names: Mazzula, Silvia L., author. | LiVecchi, Pamela, author.
Title: Ethics for counselors : integrating counseling and
  psychology standards / Silvia L. Mazzula, PhD, and Pamela LiVecchi, PsyD.
Description: New York : Springer Publishing Company, [2018] | Includes
  bibliographical references and index.
Identifiers: LCCN 2017034449 | ISBN 9780826181862
Subjects: LCSH: Counseling--Moral and ethical aspects--United States.
Classification: LCC BF636.67 .M39 2018 | DDC 174/.91583--dc23
LC record available at https://lccn.loc.gov/2017034449

> Contact us to receive discount rates on bulk purchases.
> We can also customize our books to meet your needs.
> For more information please contact: sales@springerpub.com

Printed in the United States of America.

*To Mateo, Lucas, and Xavier*
—S. L. M.

*To Nancy LiVecchi and Evelyn Oaks*
—P. L.

# CONTENTS

*Foreword, by George Stricker, PhD   ix*
*Preface   xi*
*Acknowledgments   xv*

## PART I: OVERVIEW

1. Ethics, Context, and Critical Self-Reflection   3

## PART II: MAJOR ETHICAL DILEMMAS

2. Confidentiality   19
3. Professional Boundaries   35
4. Professional Competence   49

## PART III: DYNAMIC AND CONTEMPORARY ETHICAL ISSUES

5. Culturally Competent Treatment   71
6. Managing Social Media   97
7. Confronting Colleagues and Other Sticky Situations   121

## PART IV: RECOMMENDATIONS

8. Self-Care   145
9. Counselors and Beyond   169

*Appendix   181*
*Index   183*

# FOREWORD

Ethics as an area of study has a long history dating back, in the Western world, to biblical times. It also has a short history, based on codes of ethics promulgated by professional associations. Mazzula and LiVecchi, in this practical and contemporary text, have chosen to focus on the latter, and do so in a manner that is original and timely.

There are several distinctions that must be made, and the authors address each of them. First, ethics has often been used as a synonym for anything we don't approve of. It is not unusual to hear students say, after seeing something they don't like, "That's unethical." Although something may be illegal or ill-advised, it is unethical, according to professional standards, only if it is contrary to a code of ethics. The distinction between what is illegal or ill-advised and what is unethical is a critical one, and the authors address it repeatedly and well. They continuously ask students to identify the relevant ethical issue before deciding how to act; that step is necessary and often ignored.

Codes of ethics reflect the differing domains of professional associations, and the code of the American Psychological Association (APA) and that of the American Counseling Association (ACA) differ in some trivial and some significant ways. That is a distinction I rarely see in ethics texts, and it is a centerpiece of this one. The authors present information from the standpoint of both associations, with differences pointed out clearly. It should be noted that these codes apply only to members of the relevant association, but they often are incorporated, either directly or indirectly, in licensing laws. This also leads to an important distinction. The codes apply to members of the association (or, indirectly, members of the profession) and are relevant throughout the United States (Canada has its own association and code). Laws are relevant within the state, and differ from state to state (although they do overlap, and there also are some federal statutes that apply). Thus, the ethical imperative for counselors in New York State, for example, will differ depending on whether they are licensed as psychologists or counselors, and the legal requirements will change if they should move into New Jersey or Connecticut. This can be complicated, and the text addresses the issue nicely.

Within these distinctions already discussed, there are several emergent issues, and these deserve particular attention because they often are not addressed directly by the various codes. One of these is the growing impact of social media. A counselor may be aware of many professional requirements, but not what to do about the omnipresent impact of these media. It is easy, as the codes do, to separate personal from professional accounts, but the boundaries between the two often can be fuzzy, especially given the skill some people have in evading some of the established controls. The potential benefits and disadvantages of using these media are spelled out in detail, and are necessary reading for students.

Another such contemporary area is the impact of diversity and therefore the need for cultural competence. This is not really new, as it should have been a concern for every counselor, but attention is now being given to it, and is also well developed in the text.

So far, I have indicated that the major areas of difference and value for this book are the applicability across professions and the addressing of contemporary issues. However, there is a much more important point of difference and uniqueness. An ethical decision is not simply a matter of applying a well-developed set of rules. There are many gray areas where the rules are not clear, and there is much room for individual interpretation. In order to ensure that this room for interpretation is not abused, it is critical that the counselor be sufficiently self-aware to know when individual inclinations are interfering with clear judgment. The requirement for self-awareness is described clearly and repeatedly, so that no student can come away from the text feeling that simple memorization of a code will suffice.

Self-awareness, by itself, is vital, but we are never the same from one time to another. To maintain the awareness that is so necessary, and to function at a high ethical level on a continuing basis, self-care is necessary. This too is discussed, and the student should be clear that self-awareness must be maintained and self-care is necessary for that to occur.

It is one thing to discuss these matters clearly and often, but it is another to make them living experiences for the reader. I am particularly impressed by the many ways in which the authors strive to involve the readers, whether it be by presenting dilemmas to consider or spelling out activities that highlight the points under consideration. This not only is a book that students will read with interest and enthusiasm, it also is one that will make the task of the instructor clear and easier to accomplish. I am happy to recommend it, both for students and for instructors, and look forward to its successful use.

*George Stricker, PhD*
American School of Professional Psychology
Argosy University
Northern Virginia

# PREFACE

As educators and counselors, we have worked in a variety of settings and encountered a variety of ethical dilemmas. We have both struggled to negotiate conflicts among our training models, standards of practice, workplace norms, and ethical codes. Our purpose in writing this textbook was not only to provide a nonthreatening, open environment in which to learn codes of ethics, but also to acknowledge the contextual, personal, and environmental conditions that have an impact on sound ethical decision making.

The overall goal of the textbook is to provide both counselors in training and established counselors the tools needed to make sound ethical decisions. Many of the existing educational resources focus on developing an intellectual understanding of ethical codes and standards but lack discussion of contextual and individual variables that could affect a counselor's ability to accurately perceive or respond to ethical dilemmas. *Ethics for Counselors* fills this gap.

In addition, the textbook integrates a comprehensive review of ethical standards and guidelines by two major professional governing bodies in psychology: the Ethical Principles for Psychologists and Code of Conduct of the APA, and the Code of Ethics of the ACA. Whether counselors in training learn the ethical standards and guidelines of the APA or those of the ACA depends largely on the focus of their academic program (e.g., mental health counseling terminal degrees, forensic psychology MA-to-PhD programs, clinical psychology PsyD programs), as well as the program's accrediting body. There are also students who, after receiving training under one set of ethical guidelines (e.g., ACA) at a master's level, go on to earn doctorate degrees that may transition them to use of the APA Code of Ethics. Similarly, there are counselors who were trained under one standard, but whose workplace follows the other. These situations can create a somewhat disjointed learning process, lead to difficulty managing differences in training-workplace standards, and create stressful ethical dilemmas. Thus, a key feature of this textbook is its comprehensive review of both APA and ACA ethical codes and standards, reviewing both differences and overlap.

Our approach is grounded in years of teaching students in undergraduate, master's, and doctoral-level programs, as well as clinical work with clients across the life span and in various workplace settings. We are counseling and clinical psychologists by training; therefore, each of us brings a unique clinical and professional eye regarding ethical standards that guide our professional work.

## A NOTE ON TERMINOLOGY

Throughout the textbook, we use the word *counselor*. For us, a counselor is a student, trainee, professional counselor, or psychologist who engages in therapeutic work with clients.

# LAWS AND ETHICS

Counselors must follow legal requirements and regulations that define minimum standards tolerated, which are enforced by the rule of law at the local, state, or federal level. A distinguishing feature of this textbook is its focus on engaging the reader in critically thinking through the intersections of legal requirements and ethics codes. The text guides the reader to go beyond relying solely on the rule of law, or risk-management approach, which removes the human aspect of the therapeutic relationship. However, these concepts tend to be abstract, and oftentimes confusing, especially for the developing clinician. The chapters in this textbook provide this information in a way that is straightforward, understandable, and easy to follow, using accessible lay terms.

# CRITICAL SELF-REFLECTION

A key feature of this textbook is its integration of critical self-reflection. Effective teaching of ethics needs to be done in a nonshaming way in order to increase counselors' ability to effectively recognize when they are in need of clarity or support around ethical issues. However, we recognize the tendency to, or ease with which counselors may, attribute others' ethical violations or inappropriate behavior to personality problems or intellectual deficits. We believe any counselor is capable of unethical behavior given the correct circumstances, whether they be internal (intra-psychic) or external (environmental), or both.

A distinguishing feature of this textbook is the opportunity it provides to identify variables that would place a counselor at risk. Readers are prompted to notice cognitive and emotional reactions to promote the practice of self-awareness and critical self-reflection. This, along with consistently considering contextual factors that can lead to ethical violations, will aid readers in developing the type of judgment needed to avoid ethical mishaps and develop the skills necessary for sound ethical decisions. We hope to show that making ethical decisions is more complex than following an ethical decision tree or checking off a list of ethical codes.

# ORGANIZATION OF THE BOOK

The textbook is organized in four parts:

- Part I, Overview, provides a succinct introduction (Chapter 1) to the topics discussed in detail in Parts II through IV.
- Part II, Major Ethical Dilemmas, reviews typical ethical issues that counselors encounter in practice relating to confidentiality (Chapter 2), professional boundaries (Chapter 3), and professional competence (Chapter 4).
- Part III, Dynamic and Contemporary Ethical Issues, reviews ethical dilemmas that may arise given the changing face of technology and the country's demographics relating to culturally competent treatment (Chapter 5), managing social media (Chapter 6), and confronting colleagues and other sticky situations (Chapter 7).
- Part IV, Recommendations, includes two chapters focusing on recommendations for counselors to continue sound ethical decisions (Chapters 8 and 9).

# LEARNING TOOLS

*Vignettes*: Throughout the textbook, case studies and vignettes offer opportunities for readers to practice identifying ethical dilemmas, as well as ways to proceed based on contextual variables.

*Discussion Points and Activities:* Discussion questions, self-awareness exercises, and practical activities are used to elicit in-depth exploration and practical methods for content learning and application.

*Images*: Images are strategically located to provide readers with opportunities to practice noticing personal reactions and being mindful of cognitive and emotional awareness.

*Ancillaries:* The textbook is accompanied by an instructor's manual that guides educators and supervisors through the content of the chapters, including notes for further discussion, essay questions for in-class discussion or exams, and suggested in-class activities. PowerPoints are also available. **Qualified instructors can request these ancillaries by email: textbook@springerpub.com.**

The textbook is designed for counselors in training or engaged in externships and practicums. They include master's-level students in counseling psychology, clinical psychology, and mental health programs—or other similar master's-level psychology programs—doctoral students, predoctoral students on internship, and students enrolled in programs with dual degrees (e.g., MA-to-PhD or MA-to-PsyD) or in departments that house both MA and doctoral-level programs. The book is also for established counselors who must remain abreast of changing standards and issues affecting clinical practice, such as those related to social media and technology.

For postdoctoral counselors working toward licensure, the text serves as a comprehensive resource on the ethical dilemmas and standards they need to review and the literature they need to understand in preparing for licensure exams. Lastly, the textbook serves as a resource for undergraduate-level students who are training to become Credentialed Alcoholism and Substance Abuse Counselor (CASAC), many of whom may receive in-depth training on ethical standards and on navigating ethical dilemmas by virtue of CASAC certifications being housed within undergraduate programs. Consequently, the textbook is an ideal primary text for both undergraduate and graduate-level courses in psychology, counseling, ethics, correctional studies, and training.

Some specific courses for which the book could serve as a primary or supplementary text include:

- At the graduate level:
  - Introduction to Counseling or Forensic Mental Health Counseling (primary text)
  - Ethics and the Law (primary text)
  - Practicum and Internship Seminars (primary text)
  - Theory classes such as Cognitive Behavioral Theory, Psychodynamic Theory, Integrative Psychotherapy, etc. (supplementary text)
  - Clinical courses such as Treating Addictions, Eating Disorders, Personality Disorders, and Childhood Disorders (supplementary text)
- At the undergraduate level:
  - Introduction to Counseling (supplementary text)
  - Mental Health and Ethics (primary text)
  - Theories and Interventions of Human Service (supplementary text)
  - Clinical and theory classes focused on treatment of addictions or treatment within corrections (supplementary text)

We hope you enjoy reading and working through the text as much as we enjoyed writing it. To your success.

*Silvia L. Mazzula, PhD*
*www.SilviaMazzula.com*

*Pamela LiVecchi, PsyD*
*www.PamelaLiVecchi.com*

# ACKNOWLEDGMENTS

Together we thank the staff at Springer Publishing Company, especially Sheri Sussman and Mindy Chen for their invaluable assistance, Nancy Hale (former staff) for receiving the original idea, and the creative team for designing the cover and images in this book, which help to bring the content to life. We also thank Drs. Chandler Walker, PhD, and Kelly McAleer, PsyD, for editorial services in some of the chapters.

**Silvia L. Mazzula, PhD:** I am grateful for my teachers, mentors, and scholars who have given me role models of excellent ethical judgment, self-care, and social justice. I thank the undergraduate students of my research team, especially Tiara Vega, Nathalie Velasco, and Eliza Rodriguez, who helped with references in some of our chapters—the little things that make books. I thank my friends, colleagues, and family for their support, especially my parents, Myriam and Alberto, and grandparents, Maria Esther and Abel, for teaching me that life is complex and beautiful. Lastly, and with great admiration, I thank my husband and friend, Rene, and my children, Mateo, Lucas, and Xavier, for inspiring me to do my part in making the world a better place.

**Pamela LiVecchi, PsyD:** I would like to acknowledge every teacher—and they have taken many forms throughout my life—for teaching me about compassion. Thank you, Rose and Rich, for offering the supervision and guidance that have allowed me to understand and develop my role as a professional. Most importantly, thank you to my parents, June and Joe, for being constant models for how to approach life from a place of kindness and truth. The spirit by which I approach all my work has come from both of you.

# PART I OVERVIEW

# CHAPTER 1

# ETHICS, CONTEXT, AND CRITICAL SELF-REFLECTION

Effective therapeutic services depend largely on good client–therapist relationships. Irrespective of the counselor's theoretical background, it is well documented that trust is a cornerstone of this relationship and one that is secured when counselors are able to act with excellence in professionalism and ethical behavior (Erford, 2013, 2017; Herlihy & Corey, 2006, 2015). One of the core foundations of ethical behavior is the ability to effectively navigate ethical dilemmas.

In this book, we review the ethical standards set forth by two major professional governing bodies in counseling and psychology: the Ethical Principles of Psychologists and Code of Conduct of the American Psychological Association (APA, 2017) and that of the Code of Ethics of the American Counseling Association (ACA, 2014). The book walks you through these two sets of ethical standards and discusses ethical dilemmas that cut across both APA and ACA guidelines.

There is a host of ethical dilemmas that counselors encounter. For example, dilemmas often arise related to when it is appropriate or necessary to breach confidentiality or when to refer clients when counselors exceed professional competence. In today's world of social media and technology, numerous additional ethical dilemmas arise. Should counselors be publicly present in social media platforms, or should they refrain from engaging in this dynamic and new way of communicating with the world? What if counselors witness colleagues engaging in behaviors that violate ethical standards? When and how should these be addressed, and who should do so? These are important questions that even seasoned counselors struggle with.

## INTRODUCTION TO ETHICAL STANDARDS AND GOVERNING BODIES

Ethical standards govern a counselor's professional conduct. These standards are enforced by various psychology professional organizations and state licensing boards. For counselors, these include the American Psychological Association (APA) and the American Counseling Association (ACA).

They inform how counselors engage clients, how they intervene, and how to ensure that all clients receive adequate and relevant services to address their mental health needs. These standards are outlined in APA's Ethical Principles of Psychologists and Code of Conduct (APA, 2017) and ACA's Code of Ethics (ACA, 2014).

# American Psychological Association's Ethical Principles of Psychologists and Code of Conduct

The APA code includes an Introduction, a Preamble, five General Principles (A–E), and a set of specific Ethical Standards. The Introduction, as in this textbook, talks about the intent, organization, and general scope of ethical standards. The Preamble and General Principles are aspirational in nature—that is, they provide the highest ideals that a psychologist should strive toward in the practice of psychology. Neither the Preamble nor the General Principles are enforceable rules. However, it is the intention that counselors consider these ideal behaviors when making ethical decisions. Ethical standards are enforceable rules for how psychologists should conduct themselves as professionals (APA, 2017).

# American Counseling Association's Code of Ethics

The ACA code is organized somewhat differently, yet follows a similar structure. It is organized into nine sections (A–I) and each section begins with its own Introduction, which is similar to the APA's, is inspirational in nature, and is used to guide counselors toward the highest ideals in the practice of counseling. The ACA Code of Ethics is an enforceable set of rules for how counselors should conduct themselves (ACA, 2014).

# Understanding Commonalities and Differences

In general, both sets of ethical standards are written very broadly, as to be applicable to counselors across roles and subfields. Neither set of standards is exhaustive—meaning that they do not cover every single ethical issue that may arise. However, both provide general guidance one can refer to.

You will also note that while APA makes reference to psychologists, ACA makes reference to counselors. In general, APA guides the professional practice of psychologists, whereas ACA guides the professional practice of counseling. We interpret the difference to be somewhat blurry. APA is geared more toward doctoral-level counselors and general psychology specialists. ACA, on the other hand, is geared more toward master's-level professional counselors or those in counseling fields.

Although both set of standards cover similar ethical guidelines and issues, the amount of detail given to counselors or the number of codes that inform a particularly ethical issue may vary. At times, ACA provides more detailed information or number of codes on particular issues. We find this to be related to the role of each governing body. For example, ACA appears to focus more on early career counselors or those with terminal master's degrees.

## ACTIVITY 1.1

Speak with your instructors, academic advisors, or peers about their understanding of counseling vs. general psychology fields. Does it align with your interpretation?

# RULE OF LAW AND ETHICS

Ethical issues are resolved by understanding standards that govern our professional conduct as counselors. You can find these standards in ethical codes, such as those we describe in this book (i.e., ACA or APA). There are times, however, that we encounter legal issues. These are resolved by reviewing standards that are enforced by the rule of law, at a local, state, or federal level. Laws tend to be more prescriptive than our ethical standards, although they are incorporated into ethical codes, and carry greater penalties when counselors fail to comply (Erford, 2013, 2017).

When a counselor fails to exercise "due care" in meeting professional responsibilities, he or she can be found guilty of civil liability—that is, acting wrongfully toward someone else (in this case the client) or failing to act when a counselor has the duty to act.

At various points, you will be asked to take a moment to gather the information as it relates to the specific topic of a chapter. It is really important to know that clients have the legal rights to hold counselors accountable when those clients are treated unfairly, or harmed in any way, whether it is intentional or as a result of negligence.

When clients are harmed as a result of negligence (the wrong committed by the counselor that results in injury or damage), a counselor will be held liable and sued legally through malpractice rules and procedures (Erford, 2013, 2017). Common lawsuits against counselors for negligent acts (sometimes referred as *professional negligence* or *professional malpractice*) include proving that: counselor owed a duty to the client (i.e., standards of practice), there was a breach of that duty (e.g., did not fulfill standards), and the counselor's negligence resulted in client's harm or injury in some way.

When clients are harmed as a result of an intentional act by a counselor, that counselor will be held liable and sued legally for intentional tort. Some of the common lawsuits against counselors for intentional acts include sexual assault, breach of fiduciary duty (e.g., breach of trust or confidentiality), fraud, and intentional infliction of emotional distress.

Another important concept that tends to be confusing is that of *Best Practice Guidelines*. Those are standards of practice that a counselor should strive toward and in legal proceedings are determined by testimony of peers (Erford, 2013, 2017). That means others will be called upon to testify if they would make the same choice as you did, if they were in the same situation.

Both ACA and APA have specific ethical standards regarding violations of professional conduct. For example, sexual relationship with clients is prohibited (see Chapter 3). This is a somewhat clear-cut guideline. However, sexual misconduct has been one prevalent topic in lawsuits (e.g., sexual relationships with client, sexual relationship with client's spouse, etc.). Other areas where counselors are held liable, for example, are related to breach of confidentiality or duty, exceeding professional competence, or dual relationships (e.g., see Chapter 4).

It is important not only to know the ethical standards of governing boards, but also to know state-specific laws around these ethical dilemmas. For example, in the case when a counselor has a duty to warn (i.e., must breach confidentiality), some states require the counselor to notify *either* a potential victim or the police when a client makes an explicit threat to harm a third party (note that the third party must be identifiable). Other states say a counselor has the duty to warn when the client makes an explicit threat to harm a third party (note that the third party must be identifiable) *and* the client has the intent and ability to carry out the threat. Therefore, it is critical that counselors be aware of the laws of their state. It is also important to keep up to date—that is, check regularly, as laws may change when new cases arise (see Table 1.1).

When there is conflict between ethics and the rule of law, both ACA (2014) and APA (2017) state that counselors must make known that they are committed to the ethics codes and take the steps needed to resolve the ethical dilemma. "Under no circumstances may this standard be used to justify or defend violating human rights" (APA, 1.02 Conflicts Between Ethics and Law, Regulations, or Other Governing Legal Authority). As with most ethical issues, it is always highly encouraged that counselors seek consultation. Counselors can contact professional governing boards to discuss the specific situation.

### ACTIVITY 1.2

With your supervisors and instructors, discuss the organizations and websites they use to gather information about national and state-level laws and ethical guidelines, policies, and procedures. Once you find out, write these down in a notebook for future reference. Update your notebook as new information comes up.

## THE STATE OF COUNSELOR TRAINING

Currently, when counselors are trained, they tend to learn the ethical standards and guidelines of either APA or ACA, depending on the focus of their academic program (e.g., mental health counseling terminal degree, forensic psychology MA-to-PhD programs), as well as the program's accrediting body. For example, up until recently, most doctoral and master's programs in counseling and counseling-related fields (e.g., school counseling, career counseling, additions counseling) were accredited by the Council for Accreditation of Counseling & Related Educational Programs (CACREP). CACREP-accredited programs train students to become Professional Counselors and therefore guided by the ethical standards of ACA. At the same time, we have seen an increase in academic programs that no longer seek CACREP accreditation, but are rather accredited by regional governing bodies (e.g., Masters in Psychology and Counseling Accreditation

**TABLE 1.1** Gathering Information on State, National, and Institutional Levels

### IDENTIFY ETHICAL ISSUE

Review ACA and APA codes of ethics.

- ACA Code of Ethics online: https://www.counseling.org/resources/aca-code-of-ethics.pdf
- APA Ethical Principles of Psychologists and Code of Conduct online: www.apa.org/ethics/code

Identify which ethical codes are related to your ethical dilemma.

### IDENTIFY NATIONAL RESOURCES

Locate national governing bodies that provide rules, guidelines, and ethical standards. These include, for example,

- National Board of Certified Counselors—www.NBCC.org
- American Psychological Association—www.APA.com
- American Counseling Association—www.Counseling.org
- American Mental Health Counselors Association—http://connections.amhca.org
- Association for Counselor Education and Supervision—www.acesonline.net
- Association for Multicultural Counseling and Development—www.multiculturalcounseling.org
- Masters in Psychology and Counseling Accreditation Council—www.mpcacaccreditation.org
- National Association for Addiction Professionals—www.naadac.org

### IDENTIFY STATE RESOURCES

Locate state agencies and governing boards that provide information about ethical issues and dilemmas. For example,

- State counseling ethical boards
- State psychology ethical boards
- State mental health agencies or departments

### IDENTIFY INSTITUTIONAL RESOURCES

Locate policies, procedures, and guidelines specific to your place of work. For example,

- Standard operating procedures
- Guidelines
- Polices
- Human resources

Council [MPCAC]). According to MPCAC, there were 24 accredited programs in 22 institutions across the country by the end of 2014 (Masters in Psychology and Counseling Accreditation Council, 2017).

Other non–CACREP-accredited programs may follow state guidelines or may integrate, or in some cases solely follow, the APA ethical standards and guidelines. For example, one of the institutions where we teach has a Forensic Mental Health Counseling Program. This program is a master's-level program that trains students to become professional counselors. The program is not CACREP accredited, but rather accredited through the State of New York, following the state's governing guidelines for master's-level students. Some of these students may work in traditional counseling settings, which are guided by ACA guidelines. Other students may work in general psychology-related fields at hospitals or institutions, which are predominantly guided by APA standards. Thus, students are challenged to understand not only the ethical guidelines of their training programs, but also those of their supervisions and workplace.

Similarly, there are programs with dual degrees in counseling and psychology (e.g., MA-to-PhD or MA-to-PsyD) or departments that house both MA counseling and doctoral-level psychology programs. In this trajectory, programs typically begin training students with ACA standards at the master's level and subsequently instruct them to understand APA standards upon entrance to doctoral programs. This creates somewhat fragmented learning and also poses challenges for the developing counselor.

### ACTIVITY 1.3

Explore the accreditation of your program/department. Once you find out the credentialing body, ask your instructors and supervisors which ethical standards guide their professional work.

## WHO IS THIS BOOK FOR?

## Master's- and Doctoral-Level Students

The textbook is for counselors-in-training or engaged in externships and practicums. They include master's-level students in counseling psychology, clinical psychology, and mental health programs—or other similar master's-level psychology programs. At this stage in your career development, you are training to become a licensed counselor. Depending on your program, you will be guided by different ethical standards. We hope to provide a comprehensive overview of the ACA and APA guidelines to help you navigate ethical dilemmas, which at times may seem daunting—particularly if your workplace follows a different set of standards from your program (we see this quite a bit as educators and counselors).

The textbook is also for doctoral students, predoctoral students on internship, and for students enrolled in programs with dual degrees (e.g.,

MA-to-PhD or MA-to-PsyD) or in departments that house both MA and doctoral-level programs. If you are one of these students, you may begin learning ACA standards at a master's level and—once you graduate and move on to the doctoral program—subsequently will be instructed to understand APA standards. Throughout the textbook, we try to bridge this gap for those on this academic trajectory, so that you can effectively transfer your knowledge from your MA to your doctoral training.

## Counselors

The book is also for established counselors who must stay abreast of changing standards and issues affecting clinical practice, such as those related to social media and technology. For postdoctoral counselors who are working toward their licensure, the text serves as a comprehensive resource on the ethical dilemmas and standards and other literature that they would need to review and understand for licensure exams.

## Undergraduate Students

The textbook is also a resource for undergraduate students who are training to become a Credentialed Alcoholism and Substance Abuse Counselor (CASAC). Upon graduation, bachelor-level professionals can provide direct clinical service through certifications such as the CASAC. According to the U.S. Department of Education, National Center for Education Statistics (NCES), 6% of the 1.7 million bachelor's degrees conferred between 2009 and 2010 were in psychology. Nearly 75% of undergraduate psychology degree graduates go directly into the workforce. As of September 2012, for example, there were approximately 7,063 CASACs, and 99 CASAC certification programs in New York alone (see www.oasas.ny.org). However, CASAC-eligible students are likely to receive limited in-depth training on ethical standards and on navigating ethical dilemmas, by virtue of CASAC certifications being housed within undergraduate programs. In addition, while CASAC students tend to be guided by the ethical standards of the National Association for Addiction Professionals (www.naadac.org), CASAC programs can be housed in both counseling and psychology departments. Therefore, instructors for these students vary from counselor educators (guided by ACA) to psychologists (guided by APA).

# BOOK FORMAT: OVERVIEW ON HOW TO READ IT

## General Structure

The chapters that follow are organized in three parts focusing on major ethical dilemmas (Part II), dynamic and contemporary ethical issues (Part III), and recommendations (Part IV). In each part, we provide a comprehensive overview of ethical guidelines that cut across both APA and ACA.

Each chapter, within these sections, includes case studies or vignettes to highlight the ethical issue in practice. One frustrating answer that students hear when asking about how to resolve ethical dilemmas is "it depends . . . it all depends." Cases throughout the book pose several ethical dilemmas, and arriving at a sound ethical decision depends on many factors, including, for example, the background of the client, the client's presenting problems, and the laws that guide the counselor's professional work in a given state.

In Part II, we provide instructions for methods of analyzing and working through the dilemma. After working through Part III, the reader will be prepared to take a more independent approach toward identifying the applicable ethical codes in the vignettes. However, you can read the book in the order in which the chapters are presented or read the chapter that captures your current ethical dilemma. You can switch back and forth in whatever order fits your learning style and needs.

## Part II: Major Ethical Dilemmas

In this first part of the book, we review ethical issues that consistently come up in practice. These include confidentiality (Chapter 2), professional boundaries (Chapter 3), and professional competence (Chapter 4). They are often causes for ethical violations, as noted previously. Pope and Vetter (1992) found that violations of confidentiality, dual relationships or sexual misconduct (professional boundaries), and exceeding professional areas of expertise (professional competence) are common unethical behaviors. In addition, these specific ethical guidelines are often so confusing and open to interpretation that even seasoned counselors may struggle with them.

**Chapter 2: Confidentiality** reviews ethical issues related to confidentiality. Confidentiality is a core principle with clear expectations. In general, confidentiality is the duty to keep a client's information from an unauthorized party. However, this can become difficult to apply in certain instances. For example, the requirement does not apply when disclosure is needed to protect a client or someone identifiable. For the developing counselor, and often even for seasoned counselors, it is a dilemma to determine when to breach confidentiality.

Other gray areas, for example, include issues such as dealing with life-threatening diseases that incorporate additional considerations (e.g., confirmation of diagnosis; see ACA Code B.2.b., p. 7) when determining whether breaching confidentiality is appropriate or not (ACA, 2014). Additionally, every workplace will have its own culture and standards regarding the methods used for maintaining confidentiality. Accordingly, the chapter provides guidance on comparing workplace practices with ethical standards. There are several gray areas we will review. In particular, this chapter goes over when to discuss issues of confidentiality, protecting client information from unauthorized third parties, and determining if it is important or necessary to breach one's responsibility to maintain confidentiality.

In **Chapter 3: Professional Boundaries**, we review professional boundaries, which pose similar challenges. These sets of ethical codes can seem daunting and confusing for the developing counselor, particularly within environments that create direct challenges for maintaining professional boundaries, such as correctional institutions or substance abuse clinics. Similarly, although both ACA and APA encourage clinicians to "avoid" nonprofessional relationships with current clients (e.g., going out to eat), as well as former clients or people in the client's immediate family (e.g., family members; see ACA Code, A.5.c., p. 5), others suggest that such interactions may be beneficial.

Training counselors are in a uniquely vulnerable position given the lack of professional and personal experiences, which more seasoned counselors rely on to exercise judgment. For this reason, we cover the difference between a boundary crossing and a boundary violation. In order to respect the influence of the environment on the actions of the counselor, we provide an explanation of cultural and work norms and how they can impact behavior or judgment. The chapter also reviews how the codes address self-disclosure, the receipt of gifts, and inappropriate relationships.

**Chapter 4: Professional Competence** covers the last major ethical dilemma of the first part of the book. It centers around professional competence with regard to education, training, and professional experience. For counselors-in-training, however, initial experiences are outside of their competence given their lack of clinical practice. Similarly, there may be situations in which a seasoned counselor is faced with clients who are outside of their level of competence. Counselors in these circumstances are thus required to rely properly on direct supervision and consultation, and to gain the knowledge necessary for either treating or making referrals for their clientele. This is often left up to the discretion of counselor, supervisors, and the training or work site.

An aspect discussed less, and one which students are less prepared to tackle, is that of monitoring self-impairment and effectiveness. Training counselors' initial experiences providing therapy are outside of their competence given their lack of practice. Counselors, in this circumstance, are thus required to rely on direct supervision to gain the knowledge necessary for treating their clientele, which is often left up to the discretion of the training or work site. Thus, this chapter reviews methods for recognizing the limits of one's professional competence due to training or skill, as well as recognizing one's lack of competence based on personal problems that are affecting one's ability to function effectively.

## Part III: Dynamic and Contemporary Ethical Issues

This part of the book reviews ethical guidelines surrounding dynamic and contemporary ethical issues. These include culturally competent treatment (Chapter 5), managing social media (Chapter 6), and confronting colleagues and other sticky situations (Chapter 7). With the changing demographic characteristics of our clients, the rise in technology use and often transparency of our professional and, at times, personal lives with the use of social media, these issues can become causes for ethical violations. Though some codes have clearer guidelines, others are still in development. Thus, it is often the counselor's responsibility to seek supervision and consultation in order to make ethical decisions.

In **Chapter 5: Culturally Competent Treatment**, we review ethical standards and guidelines around working with diverse populations. Multiculturalism has long been left out of mainstream psychology, training programs, and ethics. Training specific to providing culturally competent ethical decisions is often the central focus of specialized graduate programs or courses. However, incorporating cultural issues is required by ethical and credentialing bodies and has infused both ACA and APA guidelines. In fact, APA has its own publication that focuses specifically on multicultural competence along various domains, including clinical work (APA, 2002). There are several gray areas we will review in the book. In particular, this chapter covers work with diverse clients, maintenance of multicultural competence, and the role of self-awareness in the client–counselor therapeutic relationship.

**Chapter 6: Managing Social Media** discusses contemporary issues surrounding social media and its potential to create ethical dilemmas. Although both APA and ACA ethics codes provide some guidance regarding social media, it is a developing area. Professional literature regarding social media does not exist to the extent that it does in other areas. Yet, social media has become a major part of people's day-to-day activity. From our own clinical work, we know clients who have googled the names of counselors before their first session, to learn more about them. Therefore, specific training on navigating ethical issues related to social media is necessary. Specially, this chapter deals with issues related to virtual relationships, conflicts related to accurate web representation, and confidentiality.

In **Chapter 7: Confronting Colleagues and Other Sticky Situations**, we review potentially "sticky situations," such as what to do when colleagues engage in unethical behavior. There are ethical standards that provide guidelines for how one should react to a colleague who is engaged in unethical behavior. However, what is "appropriate" tends to be determined by the counselor. Furthermore, despite the clarity of expectations, responding appropriately to a colleague's unethical behavior can be challenging and confusing. Therefore, this chapter acknowledges situational variables that make this responsibility challenging, such as personal values, the relationship to the person engaging in unethical behavior, and workplace norms. This chapter reviews how to address a colleague's seemingly impaired professional competence and respond to clear violations of the ethics code.

## Part IV: Recommendations

The last part of the book focuses on counselor self-care and recommendations for moving forward with sound ethical decision-making strategies and skills. With the changing role of counselors, the shift in demographic characteristics of our clients which are often in conflict with mainstream psychology, and rise of technology, the importance of self-care has never been greater. The importance of lifelong learning and participation of supervisors and educators in the development of competent counselors is also great.

In **Chapter 8: Self-Care**, we focus on the importance of self-care in good ethical decision making. We recognize that ethical behavior relies on more than an intellectual understanding of the codes and prohibited actions. In order to recognize and properly understand ethical dilemmas, as well as options for proceeding, counselors must be skilled in recognizing their own blind spots and instances when they require assistance. We understand that self-awareness is a skill that must be developed and practiced, and is necessary for maintaining ethical and effective behavior as a counselor. Specifically, this chapter covers specific methods for maintaining a sense of self-awareness of personal health given unique work environments and stressors. There will also be final recommendations for maintaining one's health and effectiveness throughout one's career.

In **Chapter 9: Counselors and Beyond**, the book concludes with recommendations for further learning, including recommendations to counselors, supervisors, and educators, and for training programs.

## Visuals for Ethics Engagement

Throughout the book, images are incorporated to provide the reader with an opportunity to practice noticing personal reactions. The images are strategically located in areas we find are important for the reader to stop, notice his or her reactions, and take time to self-reflect in order to best understand the content presented. We integrate these images to be used as practice toward being mindful of cognitive and emotional reactions. An appendix is also offered which provides examples of cognitive and emotional reactions. Recognizing our reactions gives us a chance to slow down our thinking and consider our next decision toward sound ethical decision making.

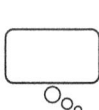

This image prompts you to engage in thoughtful *thinking and self-reflection*. This may include, for example, taking a personal inventory of your history, worldview, culture, or personal dynamics that may be affecting your experience of the information. This is not a quick process and therefore also acts a signal to slow down. In essence, the image prompts readers to put their "thinking caps" on.

As with most ethical dilemmas, there are times when so much information has to be considered that it could feel as if your brain is experiencing *information overload*. These images are located in areas where we find this to be a likely situation—not only to forewarn the reader, but also to indicate that this may be a normal reaction. This could be a result of experiencing restricted thinking or being unsure of how to think about the content. Unlike the previous image, this image highlights content that may create an impasse for counselors; it may make them feel "stuck" and, therefore, consultation may be needed.

As in most cases, resolving ethical dilemmas requires review and consultation of various sources of information. With this image, the reader is being prompted to *stop and think critically* through multiple options, ethical standards and codes, and practical ways of responding to the information presented.

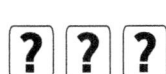

This image underscores particularly *difficult* content. The content presented may be challenging or confusing for counselors. It indicates a definite "stop" point regardless of personal reactions. It is a place to pause, digest the information, and consider multiple perspectives or ways to proceed. The reader may feel unable to think due to an intense emotional reaction.

## SELF-AWARENESS AND CRITICAL SELF-REFLECTION

A major goal when writing this textbook was to help readers tap into their thoughts, emotions, biases, and assumptions when navigating ethical standards. This provides more than a consolidation of existing codes and content. At this point in your career, we venture to say that memorizing codes is not particularly challenging. If memorization of rules was all that one needed to engage in ethical decision making, there would be no need for governing bodies to outline ethical standards and guidelines.

Therefore, we weave the human aspect of ethics throughout the text—that is, understanding ourselves, our thoughts, our emotions, and our "stuff" in ethical decision making. For example, how do our family histories, personal experiences, or social identities (e.g., racial, cultural, gender, etc.) impact how we view ethical dilemmas or how we go about making an ethical decision? Our needs, our thoughts, our reactions, and our "stuff" will inform the decisions we make.

In general, when learning about ethical decision making, counselors are often given an ethical decision-making tree, which is used as a guide to make an ethically sound decision. One such decision-making tree includes the following steps (Erford, 2013, 2017):

1. Identify the nature of the ethical dilemma. That is, what is the main problem?

2. Pick the ethical code(s) that would best help resolve the ethical dilemma you have identified.

3. Consult with colleagues or peers and standards of practice within your specialty field (e.g., school counseling).

4. Come up with a list of possible courses of action, based on your review of ethical codes and consultation with colleagues.

5. Consider the consequences of each potential course of action.

6. Arrive at a sound ethical decision.

However, arriving at sound ethical decisions must include the counselor as a key player. Pope and Vazquez (2016) discuss various other steps. Perhaps one of their major contributions is the understanding of how personal biases and assumptions impact our ethical decisions. For example, will our social identities (e.g., racial, cultural, gender, etc.) impact how we view ethical dilemmas or how we go about making an ethical decision? Our needs, our stuff, our subconscious will inform the decisions we make. Therefore, making sound ethical decisions is more than checking off or crossing out a list of codes. It is really about us as individual agents of change and how we can recognize where we might make faulty choices.

We know people do not want to break rules, especially counselors. However, one of the most important things in ethics is to understand that everyone is capable of being unethical. Recognizing the conditions under which people make wrong decisions helps our clients, ourselves, and our colleagues.

We see the development of personal growth and self-awareness as a critical and actively present aspect of ethical decision making. With this in mind, each chapter includes discussion questions that facilitate self-awareness.

# CONCLUSION

In this chapter we covered the rules and laws that govern a counselor's ethical obligations. We reviewed the variety of professionals that must adhere to these guidelines as well as the professional bodies, such as APA and ACA, that oversee these professionals. Sound ethical decision making requires an understanding of these ethical guidelines, state standards, and national standards, as well as self-awareness. You will be referred back to this chapter throughout this text in order to recall how to gather information regarding your specific laws or legal requirements. You will also be referred back to Activity 1.4 to review a self-reflection as it relates to each chapter's ethical dilemmas.

### ACTIVITY 1.4

Explore the following questions. Come back to them after you read each chapter and see if your answers change or deepen.

1. Have I engaged my own therapy and working on knowing my "stuff"? If not, would it be helpful to participate in therapy at this present time?
2. What aspects of my personality are triggered by my work?
3. How do my sociodemographic characteristics (e.g., race, culture, nationality, gender, religion, ability, etc.) impact how I interact with my clients?
4. How do my worldview and values impact how I engage with or treat my clients?
5. How do my social identities that have socially constructed power (e.g., White, heterosexual, affluent, native English speaker) impact how I engage or treat clients?
6. Am I able to remain self-aware, or have my personal or work conditions caused me to feel "shut down?"
7. Am I aware of the conditions under which my judgment might be impaired? If not, what can I do at this moment to identify those conditions?
8. Am I getting proper and effective supervision? What can I do, as an individual, to further improve my experience with supervision?

# REFERENCES

American Counseling Association. (2014). *2014 ACA code of ethics*. Retrieved from https://www.counseling.org/resources/aca-code-of-ethics.pdf

American Psychological Association. (2002). *Guidelines on multicultural education, training, research, practice, and organizational change for psychologists*.

Washington, DC: Author. Retrieved from http://www.apa.org/pi/oema/resources/policy/multicultural-guidelines.aspx

American Psychological Association. (2017). *Ethical principles of psychologists and code of conduct* (2002, amended June 1, 2010 and January 1, 2017). Washington, DC: Author. Retrieved from http://www.apa.org/ethics/code/index.aspx

Erford, T. B. (2013). *Orientation to the counseling profession; advocacy, ethics, and essential professional foundations* (2nd ed.). New York, NY: Pearson.

Erford, T. B. (2017). *Orientation to the counseling profession; Advocacy, ethics, and essential professional foundations* (3rd ed.). New York, NY: Pearson.

Herlihy, B., & Corey, G. (2006). *ACA ethical standards casebook*. Alexandria, VA: American Counseling Association.

Herlihy, B., & Corey, G. (2015). *ACA ethical standards casebook* (7th ed.). Alexandria, VA: American Counseling Association.

Masters in Psychology and Counseling Accreditation Council. (2017). *MPAC annual report: 2014*. Retrieved from http://mpcacaccreditation.org/mpac-annual-report

Pope, K., & Vazquez, M. (2016). *Ethics in psychotherapy and counseling: A practical guide*. Hoboken, NJ: Wiley.

Pope, K., & Vetter, V. (1992). Ethical dilemmas encountered by members of the American Psychological Association. *American Psychologist, 47,* 397–411. doi:10.1037/0003-066X.47.3.397

# PART II  MAJOR ETHICAL DILEMMAS

# CHAPTER 2

# CONFIDENTIALITY

Confidentiality is one of those terms that everyone knows at face value. However, the concept, when teased apart, is more comprehensive and complex than one would assume.

**Confidentiality** refers to the protection from unauthorized disclosure of information shared between a counselor and her or his client. Confidentiality is an ethical duty that is informed by ethical codes and standards of the American Psychological Association (hereafter referred to as APA; APA, 2017) and the American Counseling Association (hereafter referred to as ACA; ACA, 2014). There are a number of things that must be considered: whether confidentiality is enforceable, the limits of confidentiality, and the consequences related to violating the ethical duty to maintain confidential information. In general, counselors must protect the confidential information of their clients and disclose information only when the client provides consent or when there are legal justifications to do so.

> **CONFIDENTIALITY** - duty to protect clients from unauthorized disclosures.

Often the terms *confidentiality*, *privacy*, and *privileged communication* are used interchangeably, and this can create some confusion–not only for students, but even for seasoned counselors. Let us first go over these terms. Whereas confidentiality is the *ethical duty* that counselors have to their clients to not share the information disclosed in therapy with unauthorized parties, privacy is a *legal term* that gives clients the right to decide when or how they want to share, or not, the information they have shared with you in therapy. In contrast, *privileged communication* protects the client's privacy and confidentiality from entering into a legal proceeding—that is, from being revealed in the courts.

At the foundation of confidentiality is the trusting relationship between the counselor and her client. According to ACA (2014),

> *Counselors recognize that trust is a cornerstone of the counseling relationship. Counselors aspire to earn the trust of clients by creating an ongoing partnership, establishing and upholding appropriate boundaries, and maintaining confidentiality. Counselors communicate the parameters of confidentiality in a culturally competent manner. (ACA, 2014, p. 6)*

Seeking therapy is quite stressful for clients, whether it is mandated or self-referred. It takes courage and ability to become vulnerable in the presence of a stranger to open up to one's often hidden and deepest fears. In order for clients to open up to the process of therapy, they must trust that the counselor is competent to treat them (see Chapter 4) and also trustworthy with the information she or he will hold on their behalf.

For example, counselors must obtain permission to record sessions, to have sessions observed when in training, or to share records when the client is transferred. In essence, it is our guarantee of confidentiality that allows the therapeutic relationship to unfold. Therefore, confidentiality is arguably the most basic ingredient in successful therapeutic relationships.

This seems very simple. You just maintain confidentiality; you keep private what was shared and the relationship will flourish. Yet, many gray areas pose dilemmas for counselors. In this chapter, we cover some of the basic dilemmas that we have encountered as counselors and educators of students in the field. We engage in deep exploration on (a) how to ethically share information on behalf of your clients and when to do so, (b) how to protect client information from unauthorized third parties, and (c) limits to confidentiality. However, we recognize there are additional gray areas and dilemmas that arise in the process and some of these will come up in other chapters throughout the book.

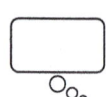

# SELF-ASSESSMENT DISCUSSION QUESTIONS: CURRENT BELIEFS AND EXPECTATIONS

## Instructions

If you were to take an essay test, how well would you be able to answer the following questions critically and thoroughly? Give yourself a letter grade from A to F. Be honest. There are no right or wrong questions when learning where you stand.

## Beliefs Regarding Confidentiality

- Role of the Counselor
  - What do you think is your role as a counselor in maintaining confidentiality? Would this be different if the client was mandated?
- Role of the Client
  - What do you think is the role of your client when it comes to confidentiality? Do you think the client should share all of his or her deepest fears with you? If so, is there a time when this is appropriate?
- Use of Confidentiality
  - In your experience, what has been the benefit of confidentiality to the client–therapist relationship? If you

have not had a formal client, can you suggest a possible benefit?
- In your experience, what has been a challenge of maintaining confidentiality in the client–therapist relationship? If you have not had a formal client, can you suggest a possible challenge?

## Expectations

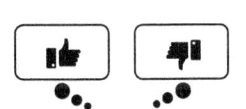

- Successes in Treatment
  - What do you think is the role of confidentiality in the success of treatment?
- Situations That May Be Challenging
  - What are two situations that might make it personally challenging for you to maintain confidentiality?
- Situations That May Create Ethical Dilemmas
  - What are two situations that would create an ethical dilemma for you when dealing with issues of confidentiality?
- Methods for Maintaining Confidentiality
  - What could you personally do to ensure the protection of your client's confidentiality?
- Impact on Self and Professional Growth
  - What is the role of confidentiality in your personal development as an individual and in your professional growth as a counselor who is continuously evolving?

# ETHICAL STANDARDS SURROUNDING CONFIDENTIALITY

First, it is important to understand where one goes to read about confidentiality in both the APA (2017) and ACA (2014) codes of ethics. Most of the codes relevant to confidentiality are grouped together. However, depending on the ethical issue you are trying to resolve, you may also see reference to confidentiality in other areas of the code of ethics. Therefore, it is important to untangle the ethical dilemma and recognize that you may need to refer to multiple codes of ethics to resolve one dilemma.

## APA Ethical Principles of Psychologists and Code of Conduct

In general, APA's standard number 4, "Privacy and Confidentiality," includes most of the confidentiality-related codes. The section starts with the principal standard, Maintaining Confidentiality (APA Code 4.01), which states:

*Psychologists have a primary obligation and take reasonable precautions to protect confidential information obtained through or stored in any medium, recognizing that the extent and limits of confidentiality may be regulated by law or established by institutional rules or professional or scientific relationship. (See also Standard 2.05, Delegation of Work to Others.) (APA, 2017)*

Following this main ethical code, APA goes on to other codes related to confidentiality, such as what to do when recording client sessions (APA Code 4.03, Recording), when disclosures are appropriate (APA Code 4.05, Disclosures), how to go about maintaining clients' privacy during consultations (APA Code 4.06, Consultations), and how to use confidential information in the case of educational activities (APA Code 4.07, Use of Confidential Information for Didactic or Other Purposes).

## ACA Code of Ethics

The ACA code discusses similar ethical standards. However, ACA dedicates a section (Section B, Confidentiality and Privacy) to discussing issues of confidentiality, beginning with an aspirational introduction that centers confidentiality in developing a trusting therapeutic alliance (see ACA, Section B, p. 6). Following this main aspirational introduction, the ACA outlines various ethical codes related to confidentiality. These include, for example, the importance of understanding how different cultures view confidentiality and privacy (ACA Code B.1.a., Multicultural/Diversity Considerations) and exceptions to confidentiality, such as when there is possible suicidal or homicidal ideation (ACA Code B.2.a., Serious and Foreseeable Harm and Legal Requirements) or end-of-life consideration (ACA Code B.2.b., Confidentiality Regarding End-of-Life Decisions), or when there are life-threatening diseases (ACA Code B.2.c., Contagious, Life-Threatening Diseases). There are also many other code portions in the ACA Code of Ethics relating to confidentiality that counselors must be aware of, such as issues of confidentiality when doing group work (ACA Code B.4.a., Group Work) or when working with couples (ACA Code B.4.b., Couples and Family).

## DIFFERENCES AND OVERLAPS

From our experience in working to make ethical decisions for the betterment of our clients, we find that ethical dilemmas often arise when we are not clear on, or there are gray areas regarding (a) when to discuss issues of confidentiality, (b) how to protect client information from unauthorized third parties, and (c) how to determine if it is important or necessary to breach our responsibility to maintain confidentiality. We review each of these dilemmas and walk through how APA and ACA can guide our ethical decisions.

### Dilemma 1: When Should Confidentiality Be Discussed?

The first dilemma is the question of when the issue of confidentiality should be discussed. Confidentiality should be addressed during the first contact with clients. This takes place during the process of obtaining informed consent, when the counselor informs the client about the therapeutic process, such as length of treatment, purpose, techniques, and potential risks (see ACA A.2.a., Informed Consent; APA, 2017). ACA includes the following in its code of ethics:

### ACA A.2.a., Informed Consent:

*Clients have the freedom to choose whether to enter into or remain in a counseling relationship and need adequate information about the counseling process and the counselor. Counselors have an obligation to review in writing and verbally with clients the rights and responsibilities of both counselors and clients. Informed consent is an ongoing part of the counseling process, and counselors appropriately document discussions of informed consent throughout the counseling relationship. (ACA, 2014, p. 4)*

APA mandates the same process, although the wording is somewhat different.

### APA 3.10 Informed Consent:

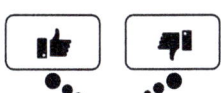

*(a) When psychologists conduct research or provide assessment, therapy, counseling, or consulting services in person or via electronic transmission or other forms of communication, they obtain the informed consent of the individual or individuals using language that is reasonably understandable to that person or persons except when conducting such activities without consent is mandated by law or governmental regulation or as otherwise provided in this Ethics Code. (See also Standards 8.02, Informed Consent to Research; 9.03, Informed Consent in Assessments; and 10.01, Informed Consent to Therapy.) (APA, 2017, p. 4)*

APA, however, is not as forthcoming about the types of information that are needed under one individual code. Therefore, counselors are charged with knowing the types of information they should share during this process. This can be particularly challenging for new counselors who must rely on standards of practice. However, APA mentions the importance of clients granting informed consent for various situations, and it does this throughout different codes in the code of ethics. For example, in the case of recording sessions, APA states:

### APA 4.03, Recording:

*Before recording the voices or images of individuals to whom they provide services, psychologists obtain permission from all such persons or their legal representatives. (See also Standards 8.03, Informed Consent for Recording Voices and Images in Research; 8.05, Dispensing with Informed Consent for Research; and 8.07, Deception in Research.) (APA, 2017, p. 7)*

In essence, both APA and ACA discuss what information counselors need to gather when it comes to informed consent. Nevertheless, counselors must be thorough in reviewing multiple codes in order to get the right information.

During informed consent, the counselor also discusses the client's rights to confidentiality, what it means for the client, and what are some exceptions to confidentiality. For example, ACA states:

### ACA A.2.b., Types of Information Needed:

*Clients have the right to confidentiality and to be provided with an explanation of its limits (including how supervisors and/or treatment or interdisciplinary team professionals are involved), to obtain clear information about their records, to participate in the ongoing counseling plans, and to refuse any services or modality changes and to be advised of the consequences of such refusal. (ACA, 2014, p. 4)*

One of these exceptions includes the involvement of supervisors (see ACA A.2.b., Types of Information Needed; APA 4.02, Discussing the Limits of Confidentiality). This is a critical part at the beginning of the professional relationship, as the client has the freedom to choose whether or not to engage in treatment with the counselor based on the information presented. In essence, informed consent gives clients the right to decide, based on the shared information, if this is something they will engage in or not.

Young counselors often believe that confidentiality is something that is only discussed at the beginning of treatment. However, informed consent is an ongoing process. Counselors are responsible for addressing this throughout the therapeutic relationship, as needed.

The issue of confidentiality also comes up throughout the therapeutic process in various instances. For example, when services are court mandated (see APA 3.10.c, Informed Consent), the client is informed at the outset about the access that the court and its representatives (e.g., probation officers) will have regarding the client's treatment. When such information is requested, counselors should discuss how information will be disclosed to ensure and safeguard a continued trusting relationship. This is critical, especially when working with criminal justice–involved clients who often feel powerless in the process. Despite the fact that, in this case, the court is the client, the person sitting in front of you also has the right to be treated fairly and to be knowledgeable about all that is happening during the treatment. We believe that even mandated clients have the right to make informed consent. That may mean discussing the pros and cons of engaging in treatment, even if mandated.

Similarly, when treating children, or adults who do not have the capacity to decide whether confidential information can be shared, counselors must (1) discuss confidentiality with said client in a developmentally appropriate way; (2) be knowledgeable about the state's age of medical consent; and (3) discuss confidentiality as often as needed or as issues arise that may require sharing of confidential information. Again, ongoing discussions will ensure that the relationship between the client and counselor is maintained and trustworthy.

## Dilemma 2: Third-Party Authorization

The second major dilemma that we can encounter concerns the release of information to third parties. In general, ACA and APA both agree that counselors must protect their client's confidential information and only release it when there are good legal or ethical reasons to do so (see ACA

B.1.b., Respect for Privacy; ACA B.1.c., Respect for Confidentiality; APA 4.04, Minimizing Intrusions on Privacy; APA 4.05, Disclosures), unless prohibited by the law. ACA codes state, for example, the following:

### ACA B.1.b., Respect for Privacy:

*Counselors respect the privacy of prospective and current clients. Counselors request private information from clients only when it is beneficial to the counseling process. (ACA, 2014, p. 6)*

### B.1.c., Respect for Confidentiality:

*Counselors protect the confidential information of prospective and current clients. Counselors disclose information only with appropriate consent or with sound legal or ethical justification. (ACA, 2014, p. 7)*

APA has very similar codes of ethics. These include, for example, the following:

### APA 4.04, Minimizing Intrusions on Privacy:

*(a) Psychologists include in written and oral reports and consultations, only information germane to the purpose for which the communication is made. (b) Psychologists discuss confidential information obtained in their work only for appropriate scientific or professional purposes and only with persons clearly concerned with such matters. (APA, 2017, p. 8)*

There are times when third parties may become involved. These include, for example: (a) when people in the client's personal life request information; (b) when a court is involved, as in the case of mandated clients; and (c) when colleagues, supervisors, or consultants are involved.

## What Happens When Others Want to Know About Our Clients?

In the case when a client would like someone to know about their treatment, whether a partner, family member, or other, the counselor cannot assume that it is acceptable to release information without the consent of the client, even if the counselor knows about this third person from conversations with the client. For example, a partner may call the counselor just to check if the client arrived at the session. This sounds like a good reason to inform the partner whether the client did or not, especially if the partner has been brought up in treatment and you know the client trusts this person. However, even if that is the case, the counselor must have written authorization to release information during the call.

Accordingly, we have made it a habit to ask clients if there is anyone they wish to share information with when we first go over informed consent. We also give examples to the client. We may ask: "Will someone be calling to see if you are here or to know if you are ready to be picked up?" If the client says yes, we ask him or her to sign an authorization to release information. We also remind clients that even if they do not have anyone at the moment, if they ever do, they must inform us and sign a release. And we explain to them that this is for their own protection.

## What Happens When the Court Is Involved?

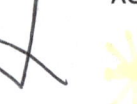

Working in the criminal justice system can cause some ethical dilemmas for even the most seasoned counselors. In a therapeutic relationship, the individual treated is the counselor's client. It is the person sitting in front of the counselor, whom the counselor is treating. However, in forensic settings (e.g., juvenile detention centers, prisons, jails, etc.), the individual treated is not the counselor's client. The client is the criminal justice system. This poses a dilemma indeed. Who then does confidentiality belong to in this case?

The criminal justice system is not designed to rehabilitate the mentally ill. Yet, since the deinstitutionalization of U.S. psychiatric hospitals, it now houses a large proportion of our mentally ill population and is the number one provider of mental health treatment. In many cases, counselors will work with a mandated client, even outside of jails or prisons.

## Counseling and the Criminal Justice System: Polar Opposite Philosophies

It is important to note here the philosophical differences of these institutions: the counseling profession (inclusive of mental health, counseling, and clinical) and the criminal justice system. A stark difference between the two is that the counseling profession focuses on respecting the client's privacy and confidentiality, whereas the criminal justice system focuses on the protection of society or that of the correctional institution.

Quite often, clients are treated as inmates first, irrespective of their mental illness, and frequently without the observance of common rights. How can we, as counselors, abide by the principle of beneficence (doing good or what is in the best interests of the "client") when we also have to protect society and maintain the status quo? As noted throughout the chapter, the counselor's work depends largely on rapport, yet clients may, directly or indirectly, question the counselor's fidelity (e.g., loyalty, faithfulness, and honoring commitments) when the counselor may be perceived as a representative of the system.

When it comes to issues of confidentiality, the court holds the client's records in literal terms. How can we, therefore, protect the client's privacy? We are also ethically bound to have our clients grant consent to treatment. However, this becomes a particularly challenging area when our clients are mandated. It is often the case that many of our ethical codes prohibit disclosure of confidential information, unless mandated by the law.

There are no clear guidelines for counselors working with clients in the criminal justice system in the context of a therapeutic relationship. ACA does state the following:

### ACA B.2.d., Court-Ordered Disclosure:

> When ordered by a court to release confidential or privileged information without a client's permission, counselors seek to obtain written, informed consent from the client or take steps to prohibit the disclosure or have it limited as narrowly as possible because of potential harm to the client or counseling relationship. (ACA, 2014, p. 7)

In some instances, institutions request that inmates sign a confidentiality form to document their understanding of the limits to confidentiality. APA has general guidelines for counselors who provide assessments or expert witness reports for clients in the criminal justice system, particularly as it relates to the importance of understanding the laws that govern their roles.

In the case of a relationship that is therapeutic in nature, it is up to the counselor to foster autonomy and agency, even when the client is mandated. It is also our utmost responsibility to follow other codes of ethics as they relate to confidentiality, so that our clients can trust us to do the work we plan to do.

## What Do We Do When Colleagues, Supervisors, and Consultations Are Involved?

Many times counselors work with others to ensure that they provide the best treatment for clients. These may be interdisciplinary teams where we present cases. Often, there are supervisors and many times experts are needed as consultants to improve services. As noted previously, the code of ethics for both APA and ACA (see ACA B.1.c., Respect for Confidentiality; and APA 4.04 b, Minimizing Intrusions on Privacy) suggests counselors may disclose information with the client's consent, when there are sound legal and ethical justifications, and only with individuals who are in some way involved with the client.

The APA has the following code regarding disclosures:

**APA 4.05, Disclosures:**

> *(a) Psychologists may disclose confidential information with the appropriate consent of the organizational client, the individual client/patient, or another legally authorized person on behalf of the client/patient unless prohibited by law. (b) Psychologists disclose confidential information without the consent of the individual only as mandated by law, or where permitted by law for a valid purpose such as to (1) provide needed professional services; (2) obtain appropriate professional consultations; (3) protect the client/patient, psychologist, or others from harm; or (4) obtain payment for services from a client/patient, in which instance disclosure is limited to the minimum that is necessary to achieve the purpose. (See also Standard 6.04e, Fees and Financial Arrangements.) (APA, 2017, p. 8)*

APA includes a similar code relating to consultations (APA 4.06, Consultations), which states the importance of maintaining the confidentiality of any information that identifies the client. ACA also includes several other guidelines regarding disclosure during case consultations in general (ACA B.7.a. and b., Case Consultation, Respect for Privacy) and as it relates to interdisciplinary teams (ACA B.3.b., Information Shared with Others, Interdisciplinary Teams).

## Sticky Conversations Outside the Office

Rarely considered as formal violations of confidentiality are conversations or consultations that often take place outside the office: for example, discussions in hallways, elevators, and even in restrooms during breaks. Although it is human nature to want to connect with others who have similar experiences, discussing client issues in public locations puts both the client and the counselor at risk.

Counselors must be aware of conditions in which they may engage in such disclosures. For example, is it stress, burnout, joy? Is it a way to relate to a colleague? A venting or informal processing session with a friend, perhaps? The role of self-awareness is critical. It is also important to keep in mind the role of self-care (see Chapter 8) and of maintaining a professional attitude at all times when it comes to discussing client issues—even if you think you left enough information out that no one would be able to identify that client.

## Dilemma 3: Exceptions to Confidentiality

The third ethical dilemma surrounds exceptions to confidentiality: that is, the limits regarding our responsibility to protect client information. As mentioned previously, APA notes psychologists recognize that "limits of confidentiality may be regulated by law or established by institutional rules or professional or scientific relationship" (APA 4.01, Maintaining Confidentiality).

In general, limits to confidentiality include cases of clients expressing suicidal or homicidal ideation and cases of abuse of children, elderly, or adults with cognitive impairment—and in some states, when clients knowingly transmit HIV. It is important to pay close attention to the key words found within our ethical codes. For example, ACA mentions that "The general requirement that counselors keep information confidential does not apply when disclosure is required to protect clients or identified others from serious and foreseeable harm . . ." (ACA B.2.a., Serious and Foreseeable Harm and Legal Requirements, p. 7). It is always good practice to consult with supervisors and colleagues when in doubt about who is considered a "client" and what it means to be "identifiable."

When counselors must breach confidentiality, it is also important to discuss this with clients, when possible. At all times, counselors must discuss limits during the informed consent conversation and at any other times when an issue may come up. Both ACA and APA have ethical codes that explain when and what information must be revealed when discussing the limits of confidentiality.

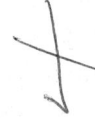

**ACA B.1.d., Explanation of Limitations:**

> *At initiation and throughout the counseling process, counselors inform clients of the limitations of confidentiality and seek to identify situations in which confidentiality must be breached. (ACA, 2014, p. 7)*

**APA 4.02, Discussing the Limits of Confidentiality:**
*(a) Psychologists discuss with persons (including, to the extent feasible, persons who are legally incapable of giving informed consent and their legal representatives) and organizations with whom they establish a scientific or professional relationship (1) the relevant limits of confidentiality and (2) the foreseeable uses of the information generated through their psychological activities. (See also Standard 3.10, Informed Consent.) (b) Unless it is not feasible or is contraindicated, the discussion of confidentiality occurs at the outset of the relationship and thereafter as new circumstances may warrant. (c) Psychologists who offer services, products, or information via electronic*

*transmission inform clients/patients of the risks to privacy and limits of confidentiality. (APA, 2017, p. 7)*

At all times, keep in mind that breaching confidentiality has the potential to create some tension for the counselor; at worst, when not done cautiously, it may lead to premature termination of the relationship. In addition to the consequences for the immediate therapeutic relationship, breaking confidentiality may create future mistrust of mental health professionals. Being aware of this, ACA encourages us to disclose only the most necessary information (ACA B.2.e., Minimal Disclosure).

### ACTIVITY 2.1

In Chapter 1, we reviewed the importance of self-awareness in arriving at sound ethical decisions. Return to Activity 1.4 and try to answer those questions as they relate to what you learned in this chapter. For example, what aspects of your personality are triggered by issues of confidentiality?

We often find it helpful to imagine others seeing our session, hearing our conversations, or reading our progress notes—remember that everything must be written. Thinking of a situation in which you would breach confidentiality, consider how you would feel if your client read the information in the progress note where you explain the information that is about to be disclosed. Now, consider how you would feel if the court read it as well. It is important both to feel good about and have a strong rationale for revealing the information you are about to disclose.

The following questions would be helpful to think through before sharing information. This also applies to sharing information via the Internet, social media, or electronic transmissions (see Chapter 6).

- Would you want your clients to see it?
    - What would it mean for them if they did?
    - What would it mean for the therapeutic relationship?
- What would happen if friends of your clients see it?
- How would you discuss this in session with your client?
- Would you need to seek supervision or consultation to competently address it with your client?
- What if a judge read it during a civil hearing or during a trial in which you were testifying as an expert?

## Engaging the Family and the Client

What helps to alleviate some of this distress is defining the limits with your client and coming to an agreement together about how to proceed. For example, there have been times when we were working with children who reported child abuse. In this case, you are a mandated reporter and must contact the appropriate authorities. Depending on institutional guidelines and state laws, you may be required to stay with the child until child protective services has been contacted and provided you with follow-up steps.

Depending on the severity of the disclosure and who the perpetrator is, we may call the caregiver to discuss what happened. We will inform them of our responsibility to call child protective services. As upsetting as this may be, we can do so in a way that engages the caregiver in resolving this problem. We may be able to ask the caregiver to come to the office so that we can call child protective services together, if the caregiver is not the perpetrator and we believe the caregiver has the child's best interest in mind. We can also frame the call as something that will provide the family with additional services, rather than a way to "rat out" the family, which at times has been our clients' perceptions.

This has worked for us in that it gave the nonoffending caregivers a chance to be part of the solution—even if the end result to call child protective services was already determined and that caregiver was so informed. We do this thinking of the child. We do this thinking of our role in making sure that we remain much a part of the relationship as possible and that the relationship does not terminate due to our breach of confidentiality.

We have taken a very similar approach in the case of suicidal ideation. We always make sure to discuss each step with our client, and in some instances, when feasible, we will accompany our clients to the hospital. We do not, however, engage our clients as a way to change our mind about the course of action we plan to take if there is reasonable cause to believe that the client is at risk. We do this as a way to engage them and to be transparent. Remember, in many states, you are required to breach confidentiality when these issues come up—but we can do so in a way that does not sever our trusting relationship. We always do follow-up sessions to discuss what happened and how the client felt in the process.

ACA goes further to provide additional and specific codes regarding limits of confidentiality. These include, for example, additional information that is needed when dealing with end-of-life decisions (ACA B.2.b., Confidentiality Regarding End-of-Life Decisions) and when there is a contagious and life-threatening disease (ACA B.2.c., Contagious, Life-Threatening Diseases). Some of these codes leave a lot to the counselor's discretion. Therefore, it is always important to engage in consultation to make the best ethical decision. At all times, counselors must be aware of the state laws regarding disclosure status, which may vary by state.

## ACTIVITY 2.2

Explore the laws in your state. Investigate whether these are in line with the ethical standards you learned in this chapter, or if they are in conflict with one another. (See Chapter 1, Table 1.1, on gathering information in your state.)

## CASE STUDY VIGNETTE

### Instructions

Following the case study vignette, we will walk through some questions on how to make an ethical decision to resolve this dilemma. Monitor your reactions to this vignette and the events that take place within it. In monitoring your reactions, keep track of any that include shaming the counselor for "bad" behavior or for being a "bad counselor." Focus on the internal and external factors that may have led to this behavior. Now is the time to notice if there are any patterns in your reactions, or the substance of your reactions, and to discuss these in supervision and consultation. This is valuable information for your reflection on what some of your personal biases and blind spots may be. (See the Appendix, Typical Cognitive and Emotional Reactions, at the end of this book.)

### Case Study

*John, an upper-class African American male, is a graduate-level student (50 credits) in a mental health* **counseling** *program. He is doing his externship at a correctional facility and has been asked to conduct an intake screening of Gloria, a new inmate. This is the information John receives before the intake. After the intake session, John may provide counseling to Gloria to accumulate his clinical hours, or he may refer her to another counselor for treatment.*

Gloria was referred for an intake interview to assess risk level and services she would need. Prior to her arrest, she had attempted suicide by overdosing on pills while in the presence of her children. Gloria is a 35-year-old, light-skinned Latina women, born in Argentina, who came to the United States when she was 18 years old. Her preferred language is Spanish, though she can communicate in English. Gloria is married to a self-identified Afro-Latino, born in Colombia, South America. Gloria and her husband met when she first arrived in the United States. They have two young children.

According to her records, Gloria has a history of sexual and physical abuse as a child by members of her family. Her history of suicide ideation dates back to when she was 8 years of age (i.e., she cut her wrists at 8 years old, wanted to jump in front of a train at 12, and tried to overdose on pain killers at 16 years of age). Gloria's history is also positive for violence toward others. At 10 years of age, she attempted to stab a classmate and at 16 she pushed her father into a running vehicle. Most recently, at 34 years of age, she was arrested subsequent to a physical altercation with a neighbor. Gloria is currently at the women's correctional facility for a violent offense. Her records note that she reported the most recent physical altercation (which resulted in her arrest) was a result of "being tired of my neighbor calling me spic and telling me to go back to my country." Her records further note that Gloria is not interested in therapy, saying "*asi es la vida* (this is life), and there is nothing I can do about it" in reference to her emotional problems. Gloria is currently in prison for a violent offense and her release day is unclear.

*(continued)*

## CASE STUDY VIGNETTE (continued)

### Resolving the Ethical Dilemma

Think about the following questions. Write your answers down before moving on to the discussion.

1. What is the ethical dilemma in this case?
2. Based on the review of ACA and APA codes of ethics throughout the chapter, which ethical code(s) should John consult to resolve this dilemma?
3. Should John seek consultation before conducting the intake interview? Or should he conduct the intake and gather more information?
4. If John decides to proceed with conducting the intake interview, what aspects of informed consent should he review with Gloria?

Now that you have written down your answers, let us go together through what John should do.

First, John should think about the ethical dilemma. What did you think it was? This seems to be a very complicated case. Gloria appears to have a long-standing history of suicidal ideation and violence attempts. Therefore, the issue of whether he should breach confidentiality seems to be the most pressing.

John decides to conduct the intake session and gather more information to determine if he should consult with his supervisor. As a student, he reviews the ACA Code of Ethics, which states that confidentiality is not "required to protect clients or identified others from serious and foreseeable harm" (ACA B.2.a., Serious and Foreseeable Harm and Legal Requirements). Knowing this, John proceeds to gather more information from Gloria to determine the severity of her suicidal ideation. Gloria reported that her last attempt was 3 years ago. She mentions that she has not felt like hurting herself since then. She also has not felt like hurting her children or her husband. Therefore, John makes note of this in his record and proceeds with the intake assessment.

When going over informed consent with Gloria, John struggles with how much time he should spend on it, since she is a mandated client. In essence, he knows her records belong to the criminal justice system and that she has little say in what will happen in treatment. However, as a competent counselor in training, John goes over the details of the informed consent (e.g., APA 3.10, Informed Consent). He includes the basic information, such as length of treatment, his approach, and his qualifications to treat her. John also tells Gloria about his student status and the fact that there will be supervisors involved in the treatment (e.g., ACA B.7.b., Case Consultation, Disclosure of Confidential Information).

Another ethical dilemma, though not related to confidentiality, is John's level of competence to treat this client. There are boundaries to competence that John should be aware of. In general, competence is based on one's education, training, experience, and credentials. What kinds of training, experience, and credentials would he need? Competence is also based on knowing the values, assumptions, and worldviews of our clients and ourselves. How can John know whether he is maintaining his level of competence is this area? (See Chapters 4 and 5 to help resolve these additional dilemmas.)

*(continued)*

### CASE STUDY VIGNETTE (continued)

#### Case Study Discussion Questions

1. What would you have done differently or the same?
2. What should John do to make sure things go well with Gloria and ensure that she engages in treatment?
3. Which gray areas were presented in this case, but not discussed, that could bring up additional ethical dilemmas?
4. Which actions within this vignette are important to note in order to best understand this situation?

# CONCLUSION

In this chapter, we covered the importance of protecting clients' privacy and confidentiality in order for the therapeutic relationship to flourish. However, we went over gray areas that pose dilemmas for counselors: (a) how to ethically provide information for your clients and when to do so, (b) how to protect client information from unauthorized third parties, and (c) what are the limits to confidentiality. Although we did not go over every code of ethics that discusses confidentiality, it is clear that one must refer to multiple codes and standards, even within one set of guidelines, in order to make an ethical decision regarding confidentiality.

In addition, always remember to know the laws regarding confidentiality. As you may recall from Chapter 1, there are different requirements, for example, based on the state where you work. Keeping up to date on laws and workplace policies and guidelines is very important.

### PERSONAL INVENTORY: QUESTIONS FOR FUTHER EXPLORATION

# PROFESSIONAL EXPERIENCES

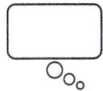

1. Can you think of a time when you struggled with determining how to protect your client's confidential information? What did you do?
2. Have you ever felt uncomfortable when a colleague was talking about a client in your presence? What did you do?
3. What are some steps that I could follow in order to determine whether or not I may be at risk of breaching confidentiality?
4. What may be some blind spots that I have regarding issues of confidentiality?
5. How can I best integrate my ethical guidelines when working in professional settings that follow a separate set of ethical standards (i.e., ACA vs. APA)? How can I ensure that I stay true to my professional identity?

## PERSONAL EXPERIENCES

1. Has there been a situation when you told someone something private with the hope that it would stay between you and them and they shared it with someone else? How did that feel?
2. Has a family member or friend ever told you a secret that you felt had to be shared? How did you go about resolving this?

## FURTHER LEARNING AND SUGGESTED READINGS

American Psychological Association. (2003). *Guidelines on multicultural education, training, research, practice, and organizational change for psychologists.* doi:10.1037/0003-066X.58.5.377

American Psychology-Law Society. Specialty Guidelines for Forensic Psychology. Retrieved from http://www.apadivisions.org/division-41/about/specialty/index.aspx

Packer, I. K. (2008). Specialized practice in forensic psychology: Opportunities and obstacles. *Professional Psychology, Research and Practice,* 39(2), 245–249.

## REFERENCES

American Counseling Association. (2014). *2014 ACA code of ethics.* Retrieved from https://www.counseling.org/resources/aca-code-of-ethics.pdf

American Psychological Association. (2017). *Ethical principles of psychologists and code of conduct* (2002, amended June 1, 2010 and January 1, 2017). Retrieved from http://www.apa.org/ethics/code/index.aspx

# CHAPTER 3

# PROFESSIONAL BOUNDARIES

The concept of boundaries is understood as a method of maintaining professional roles within the context of providing services. The intention of professional boundaries is to maintain a healthy and trusting relationship between the professional and the client. In this chapter, we address three areas that are rich with ethical dilemmas. First, it is important to establish an understanding of boundary crossings and boundary violations.

**Boundary crossings** can be seen as effective methods for building rapport, providing comfort, and in general, being flexible in order to meet clients "where they are." If boundaries represent literal and emotional spaces around us, then boundary crossings represent instances in which the counselor crosses specific personal or professional limits. When a counselor extends the length of the session in order to accommodate a client who arrived late to the session, it crosses a boundary. There is a boundary around the time and length of sessions and it was "crossed" by the therapist by allowing the session to continue past the allotted time. When counselors share a personal experience that relates to the client's experience, they have crossed a boundary. A boundary existed around what information was shared and what was kept personal, and the therapist crossed the boundary by sharing personal information. In both of these instances, the crossing is not necessarily wrong or unhealthy.

Many seasoned counselors thoughtfully and purposefully cross boundaries, in accordance with their therapeutic orientation and goals for treatment. Clinical supervisors who engaged in positive boundary crossing with trainees were viewed by the trainees as enhancing the supervisory experience or the clinical training experience (Kozlowski, Pruitt, Dewalt, & Knox, 2014). Many new counselors may cross boundaries in an attempt to build rapport or as a result of lack of judgment. When counselors cross boundaries, they should be doing so for a purpose and in a way that is supportive of a healthy therapeutic relationship.

Counselors hold the responsibility for maintaining safety within the therapeutic relationship, and it should be noted that most of our information regarding the experience of boundary crossings has come from the perspective of the counselor (Fasasi & Olowu, 2013). Therefore, seeking consultation and supervision regarding any boundary crossings is recommended. There are major differences between boundary crossings, which can be useful, and boundary violations, which are hurtful.

**Boundary violations** can include engaging in a romantic relationship with a client, working in some other professional capacity with a client (e.g., employment), or treating a close family member or friend of a client.

Boundary violations are seen as harmful to the client and the effectiveness of the therapeutic relationship. These violations can lead to disciplinary actions from the state licensing board, as well as civil lawsuits from the licensing board and/or the client/patient in question. In 2010, 30% of the ethics complaint cases that were opened by the American Psychological Association (APA) were for "dual relationships" which included sexual misconduct, sexual harassment, or nonsexual dual relationships (Anderson, 2011).

According to a well-known survey of members of APA conducted by Pope and Vetter (1992), 17% of reported dilemmas dealt with blurred, dual, or conflictual relationships. Boundary violations often begin as boundary crossings. The path toward boundary violations has been referred to as the *slippery slope*. This includes multiple actions within a seemingly gray area, that are not acknowledged by the counselor as inappropriate, may be rationalized, and lead to a boundary violation which is no longer within a gray area. What are often viewed as *gray areas* with regard to boundaries can be understood as the space between a rigid adherence to a boundary and a boundary violation. It is important to recognize this space. This gray area can be thoughtfully managed to the benefit of the client/patient, or can be the beginning of a "slippery slope" toward a boundary violation, which will inevitably harm the counselor.

> **BOUNDARY CROSSING** - Instance in which the therapist crosses specific personal or professional limits without engaging in an ethical violation.
>
> **BOUNDARY VIOLATION** - Instance when a counselor crosses a boundary in a way that is harmful to the client, is in violation of the ethics code, and may result in disciplinary action by a state or national organization.

Maintaining boundaries can be challenging for a variety of reasons. It is important to understand some of the variables that impact our individual understanding and application of boundaries within therapeutic relationships. In practice, maintaining boundaries relies on our interpretation of the situational application of principles and standards. Counselors may avoid acknowledging or sharing certain feelings about clients because of fear or shame. However, feelings alone do not cause behavior. For example, whereas there may be many counselors who have had sexual feelings about clients, few actually engage in sexual activity with clients, which would clearly be a violation of ethical standards (Pope, Sonne, & Greene, 2006). It is essential that counselors begin to acknowledge the role that multiple internal (intrapsychic) and external (environmental) variables can have on their behavior. Reviewing variables that we should all be aware of when understanding our reactions to this work is important.

# CULTURAL NORMS, INTERNAL DYNAMICS, AND WORKPLACE NORMS

Cultural norms regarding boundaries, internal dynamics, and workplace norms all impact a person's sense and application of boundaries.

A multitude of cultural norms or variables impact a person's sense of boundaries; these variables include a person's family background, as well as the immediate culture in which he or she lives. Certain cultures promote physical touch and emotional expression more than others. Some cultures are more comfortable with sharing personal information or sharing gifts. Our culture-bound perception of maintaining boundaries, while preserving a therapeutic relationship, affects our choices to accept gifts or hug a client, for example; this perception even affects our basic physical behavior, such as how close we sit to a client in the office.

There are intercultural differences in *personal space* (Beaulieu, 2004), which is a construct that is developed in relationship to the environment and depends on culture. Personal space is a clear example of expectations and potentially a source of misunderstanding. Specific cultural variables can influence a counselor's resolution of ethical issues (Zheng, Gray, Zhu, & Jiang, 2014). Counselors are tasked with having sufficient understanding of how their culture impacts their view on boundaries. This is not necessarily an easy task. Reflecting on one's own culture often requires outside assistance, such as counseling or supervision. Lacking an appreciation for one's cultural expectations regarding boundaries can have serious consequences, such as misjudging what is appropriate within a therapeutic relationship or misunderstanding a client's behavior. (See Chapter 5, "Culturally Competent Treatment.")

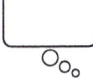

In addition to cultural norms, internal dynamics or personality greatly affect an individual's experience of boundaries. Our personalities intersect with cultural variables and motivate our behavior within relationships. If cultural norms impact our perception of our behavior and that of others, personality can be seen as an even more fundamental filter through which we see the world. Personality is our expectation of ourselves and others; our sense of consistency and safety, and our sense of autonomy that impacts how we view and relate to others. From that standpoint, a core component of relationships is setting boundaries. Boundaries, which represent a space or limit between people, serve to maintain a sense of safety, autonomy, and respect. Lacking an appreciation for how one's personality is impacting one's behavior within relationships could have serious negative consequences.

Separate, but possibly related, is the counselor or psychologist's mental health, which can directly impact the boundaries within a therapeutic relationship. This can include bouts of anxiety or depression, issues within relationships, or substance abuse. As our internal experience shifts, so may our interaction with our work. When counselors engage in unethical behavior with clients, the responsibility falls on the counselor and may have been the result of internal difficulties that were not properly addressed or managed. Although some may identify the profile of a client who may put a counselor at risk for a boundary violation, there is no single profile of a client who is the victim of a sexual relationship with their therapist (Celenza, 2007). As it is the "fault" of the counselor, we must be aware of what may impact a counselor's ability to uphold ethical standards. The mental health of the counselor is addressed through APA Code 2.06, Personal Problems and Conflicts, which states:

*(a) Psychologists refrain from initiating an activity when they know or should know that there is a substantial likelihood that their personal problems will prevent them from performing their work-related activities in a competent manner. (b) When psychologists become aware of personal problems that may interfere with their performing work-related duties adequately, they take appropriate measures, such as obtaining professional consultation or assistance, and determine whether they should limit, suspend, or terminate their work-related duties. (See also Standard 10.10, Terminating Therapy.) (APA, 2017, p. 5)*

The American Counseling Association (ACA) addresses the interaction between the counselor's personal values and work through Code A.4.b., Personal Values, which states: "Counselors are aware of their own values, attitudes, beliefs, and behaviors and avoid imposing values that are inconsistent with counseling goals. Counselors respect the diversity of clients, trainees, and research participants." ACA also addresses the counselor's mental health through Code C.2.g., Impairment, which states:

*Counselors monitor themselves for signs of impairment from their own physical, mental, or emotional problems and refrain from offering or providing professional services when impaired. They seek assistance for problems that reach the level of professional impairment, and, if necessary, they limit, suspend, or terminate their professional responsibilities until it is determined that they may safely resume their work. . . . (ACA, 2014, p. 9)*

The code goes on to state that counselors should assist colleagues with recognizing their impairment (see Chapter 4).

Managing boundaries is particularly challenging within certain work environments. Workplace norms, which are standard actions and patterns that occur within a specific workplace, determine acceptable and unacceptable behaviors. Psychiatric hospitals, correctional institutions, substance abuse treatment centers, and private practices all have their own unique norms for employee behavior. For example, a workplace norm within a substance abuse treatment center may be for the counselors to disclose their history with substance abuse and recovery. Although there may be no written rules in the employee manual dictating that they do so, new employees will see that most counselors are discussing their histories with substance abuse and recovery and that most clients are expecting their counselors to share this information. There are pros and cons to this type of disclosure. However, regardless of the incoming counselors' views on this type of self-disclosure, they will likely experience the pull to follow the norm; if they do not, they may experience a sense of disconnection from the rest of the staff, and possibly the clients, for breaking with the norm. Other workplace norms may include methods for interacting with clients and methods for communication among staff. Important to note are workplace norms regarding the openness of counselors with regard to questions or concerns they have.

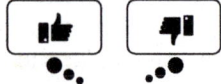

There are many ethical dilemmas related to maintaining healthy boundaries. Maintaining boundaries with clients should be at the forefront of a clinician's mind throughout her or his career and should be reviewed regularly depending on the client, their work environment, and their personal reactions to clients. In this chapter, we focus on three typical dilemmas that occur within counseling relationships: (a) self-disclosure, (b) accepting gifts, and (c) inappropriate relationships. We review each of these dilemmas and walk through how the APA's Ethical Principles of Psychologists and Code of Conduct and the ACA's Code of Ethics can guide our ethical decisions.

### ACTIVITY 3.1

In Chapter 1, we reviewed the importance of self-awareness in arriving at sound ethical decisions. Return to Activity 1.3 and try to answer those questions as they relate to what you learned in this chapter. For example, what aspects of your personality are triggered by certain client/patient characteristics, such as personality traits, or situational variables?

## SELF-ASSESSMENT: CURRENT BELIEFS AND EXPECTATIONS

### Instructions

If you were to take an essay test, how well would you be able to answer the following questions critically and thoroughly? Give yourself a letter grade from A to F. Be honest. There are no right or wrong answers when "learning where you stand."

### Beliefs

- Role of the Counselor
  - What do you think is the role of a counselor in maintaining professional boundaries? You may think of what your role does and does not consist of, as well as what you believe your responsibilities are.
- Role of the Client
  - How do you think a patient or client plays a role in maintaining professional boundaries?
  - What are your expectations of how a client of yours should and should not behave regarding the boundaries between you?
- Function of Boundaries
  - What may be some benefits of maintaining professional boundaries in a client–therapist relationship?
  - How do you think boundaries could support the therapeutic relationship or the client's progress?

## ACTIVITY 3.2

Explore what successful treatment looks like for you and your clients. Is it low turnover rate, good rapport, or long-term engagement? How would you know if your treatment was successful? Could you measure it?

## Expectations

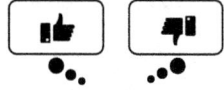

- Successes in Treatment
  - What do you think is the role of boundaries in the success of treatment?
- Situations That May Be Challenging
  - In general, which types of situations or environments could be challenging for maintaining your role as a counselor?
  - What factors may challenge the boundaries within a client–counselor relationship?
  - What cultural or situational variables may create a challenge for maintaining the types of boundaries you believe you should be maintaining?
- Situations That May Create Ethical Dilemmas
  - What are two situations that would *likely* create an ethical dilemma for you when dealing with issues related to boundaries?
  - Think of yourself, specifically: What is it about your experience with boundaries and relationships that would likely impact your thinking and behavior within the context of treatment?
- Methods for Maintaining Boundaries
  - What do you actually do to maintain boundaries? Think of actions, as well as inner processes that the client may not see.

# REVIEW OF ETHICAL STANDARDS SURROUNDING BOUNDARIES

First, it is important to understand where one can read about professional boundaries in both codes of ethics. Both APA and ACA approach the issue of boundaries differently. Depending on the ethical issue you are trying to resolve, you may also see references to professional boundaries in other areas of the code of ethics. Therefore, it is always important to untangle the dilemma and recognize the need to refer to multiple codes of ethics.

## APA Ethical Principles of Psychologists and Code of Conduct

In general, boundaries are not addressed independently of other topics within the APA ethics codes, meaning that there is not a "boundaries" section or separate standard that describes what they are and how they should be applied. Instead, boundaries are directly or indirectly addressed through the standards for maintaining professional boundaries, by avoiding multiple relationships, respecting our boundaries of competence, and by upholding appropriate boundaries within a therapeutic relationship.

## ACA Code of Ethics

The ACA ethics code addresses boundaries on their own and within other various codes. Professional boundaries are also related to other ethical standards, such as confidentiality. The ACA code directly states that confidentiality is dependent on upholding professional boundaries, as well as maintaining appropriate boundaries within the supervisory relationship.

## DIFFERENCES AND OVERLAP

In this chapter, we focus on three typical dilemmas that occur within counseling relationships: (a) self-disclosure, (b) accepting gifts, and (c) inappropriate relationships. We review each of these dilemmas and walk through how APA and ACA can guide our ethical decisions. The appropriate, the inappropriate, and the gray areas: What are they and how can we tell?

## Dilemma 1: Self-Disclosure

**Self-disclosure** is an easy way to explore gray areas within the therapeutic relationship. If "privacy is viewed as a process of boundary regulation, controlling how much (or how little) contact an individual maintains with others" (Derlega & Chaikin, 1977, p. 102), then what is self-disclosure? Regarding the "norms" previously mentioned in this chapter, self-disclosure, and what is expected of the counselor in that respect, may vary depending on the environment. Properly, *self-disclosure* is defined as "a conscious, intentional technique in which clinicians share information about their lives outside the counseling relationship" (Simone, McCarthy, & Skay, 1998, p. 174). Self-disclosure may include sharing if the counselor has children, the area in which she lives, or information relating to his daily life. There are unintentional disclosures, such as the therapist's age or gender, which can just be observed by the client. However, here we are talking about the counselor actively participating in sharing personal information. This could be useful for building rapport or normalizing the client's behavior. Understanding when self-disclosure is appropriate or not depends on the environment (corrections vs. private practice), as well as the dynamics in the therapeutic relationship.

Although this may appear straightforward, understanding self-disclosure could become complicated and become a gray area. The appropriateness of self-disclosure could be understood by referring to APA codes, such as 3.04, Avoiding Harm, or 3.05, Multiple Relationships, but self-disclosure itself is not directly or specifically addressed in the code. In these cases, it may be most useful to refer to the principles for assisting in decision making.

Similarly, ACA does not give specific direction regarding clinician self-disclosure, so we are required to refer to codes such as A.1.a., Primary Responsibility, which states "The primary responsibility of counselors is to respect the dignity and to promote the welfare of clients" (ACA, 2014, p. 4), and A.4.a., Avoiding Harm, for guidance.

> **SELF-DISCLOSURE** - The counselor's intentional or active sharing of personal information with a client.

### How Can We Tell What's Healthy or Appropriate?

The easiest way to tell if a behavior is healthy and appropriate vs. unhealthy and inappropriate is to gain an objective opinion regarding your actions and how they match up with the ethics code. Many times, counselors share personal information in an attempt to reduce their own anxiety, along with the client's. Supervision and consultation are effective for understanding the true motives for self-disclosure. Gaining an initial opinion from someone who is not motivated to simply agree with your behavior can be an effective tool for receiving feedback.

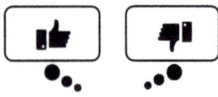

Would you rather figure out this counseling-related issue on your own because you are worried about how your colleague or supervisor may respond? Well, that is actually a strong indicator that you require assistance with reviewing your actions and motivations for your behavior. The saying goes: "If you think it is something that you would like to hide from your supervisors, then that is exactly the thing that you should be sharing with them."

It is important to note that any counselor is at risk of engaging in a boundary violation under certain circumstances, such as when dealing with large life stressors or mental health impairment. It is uncomfortable to acknowledge, but given the right conditions, we are all capable of unprofessional behavior. Although there may be profiles of counselors who act inappropriately, it is most important to remain aware that anyone is capable of a misstep so that we quickly recognize our own.

## Dilemma 2: Accepting Gifts

During the course of treatment, or at the point of treatment termination, clients may offer the therapist a gift as a symbol of appreciation. This creates an interesting dilemma, since many variables could be considered in order to determine if accepting the gift could harm the client. Variables could include: the cost or value of the gift, the point in therapy at which the gift is being offered, and what the gift symbolizes to the client. APA does not directly discuss taking gifts within the standards. However, one could refer to APA's Principle A of "doing no harm," and consider cultural context, in order to determine the impact of taking a gift. In this case, the counselor needs to understand that taking gifts should be decided based on this principle. In contrast, ACA does directly address taking gifts from clients. ACA Code A.10.f., Receiving Gifts, states:

*Counselors understand the challenges of accepting gifts from clients and recognize that in some cultures, small gifts are a token of respect and gratitude. When determining whether to accept a gift from clients, counselors take into account the therapeutic relationship, the monetary value of the gift, the client's motivation for giving the gift, and the counselor's motivation for wanting to accept or decline the gift. (ACA, 2014, p. 6)*

## Dilemma 3: Inappropriate Relationships

Although neither APA nor ACA provides a specific section for understanding professional boundaries, both include sections that address methods for maintaining healthy and appropriate behaviors within the therapeutic relationship. We can also rely on the General Principles as a guide for resolving ethical dilemmas that are not addressed directly through each standard's individual codes. APA's Standard 3, Human Relations, and Standard 10, Therapy, provide guidance for ways to avoid harm and inappropriate relationships with past or current clients. Section A in the ACA code, titled "The Counseling Relationship," contains codes that address the issue of boundaries.

Within the realm of boundaries, both the APA and ACA codes agree that romantic relationships with past or current patients are harmful. APA Code 10.06, Sexual Intimacies with Relatives or Significant Others of Current Therapy Clients/Patients, prohibits "sexual intimacies with individuals they know to be close relatives, guardians, or significant others of current clients/patients" and states "Psychologists do not terminate therapy to circumvent this standard" (p. 14). APA Code 10.07, Therapy with Former Sexual Partners, prohibits accepting a former sexual partner as a therapy patient, and APA Code 10.8, Sexual Intimacies with Former Therapy Clients/Patients, prohibits sexual relationships with former patients for at least two years following the cessation of therapy—nd even then, only within "the most unusual circumstances." The code reads:

> *(a) Psychologists do not engage in sexual intimacies with former clients/patients for at least two years after cessation or termination of therapy.*
> *(b) Psychologists do not engage in sexual intimacies with former clients/patients even after a two-year interval except in the most unusual circumstances. Psychologists who engage in such activity after the two years following cessation or termination of therapy and of having no sexual contact with the former client/patient bear the burden of demonstrating that there has been no exploitation, in light of all relevant factors, including (1) the amount of time that has passed since therapy terminated; (2) the nature, duration, and intensity of the therapy; (3) the circumstances of termination; (4) the client's/patient's personal history; (5) the client's/patient's current mental status; (6) the likelihood of adverse impact on the client/patient; and (7) any statements or actions made by the therapist during the course of therapy suggesting or inviting the possibility of a posttermination sexual or romantic relationship with the client/patient. (See also Standard 3.05, Multiple Relationships.) (APA, 2017, p. 15)*

There is a difference between the APA and ACA codes regarding the specifics of sexual relationships with former clients. The ACA code is consistent with the APA code, as demonstrated by ACA Code A.5.a., Current Clients, which prohibits "[s]exual or romantic counselor–client interactions or relationships with current clients, their romantic partners, or their family members." The ACA code differs from the APA code, as demonstrated in Code A.5.c., Sexual and/or Romantic Relationships with Former Clients, which states:

> *Sexual and/or romantic counselor–client interactions or relationships with former clients, their romantic partners, or their family members are prohibited for a period of 5 years following the last professional contact. This prohibition applies to both in-person and electronic interactions or relationships. Counselors, before engaging in sexual and/or romantic interactions or relationships with former clients, their romantic partners, or their family members, demonstrate forethought and document (in written form) whether the interaction or relationship can be viewed as exploitive in any way and/or whether there is still potential to harm the former client; in cases of potential exploitation and/or harm, the counselor avoids entering into such an interaction or relationship. (ACA, 2014, p. 5)*

In summary, both the APA and ACA codes provide guidance for managing boundaries by directly addressing some issues such as romantic relationships with clients. APA and ACA differ with regard to directly addressing issues such as receiving gifts, and neither the APA nor the ACA codes specifically address the issue of self-disclosure. Given these differences, it is recommended that you refer to whichever code applies to your specific license. For those who follow the APA or ACA code, referring to the sections that address avoiding harm assists with navigating ethical dilemmas that seem to fall within gray areas or are dictated by more than one code.

## ACTIVITY 3.3

Explore any rules of your workplace or school regarding any of the dilemmas listed in this chapter or boundaries in general. Investigate whether these are in line with the ethical standards you learned in this chapter, or if they are in conflict with one another.

## CASE STUDY VIGNETTE

### Instructions

Following the case study vignette, we will walk through some questions on how to make an ethical decision to resolve the dilemma posed therein. Remember to monitor your reactions, keeping track of any that include shaming the counselor for "bad" behavior or for being a "bad counselor." Focus on the internal and external factors that may have led to this behavior. Now is the time to notice if there are any patterns in your reactions, or the substance of your reactions, and to discuss these in supervision and

*(continued)*

## CASE STUDY VIGNETTE (continued)

consultation. This is valuable information for your reflection on what some of your personal biases and blind spots may be. (See the Appendix, Typical Cognitive and Emotional Reactions, at the end of this book.)

### Case Study

*Grace is working at a halfway house (transitional housing) for adult women who have recently been released from prison. The program provides substance abuse treatment and parenting support, as well as help with promoting healthy lifestyles for the clients upon their release.*

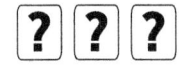

Grace is working with Nicole, an African American woman in her early 30s who is diagnosed with generalized anxiety disorder. Nicole is finishing her 8-year sentence for possession and distribution of illegal drugs. She has three children who are living in foster care. She has contact with her elderly mother and minimal contact with the rest of her family. Upon her release from this program, Nicole plans on attaining housing and regaining custody of her children. Nicole has a long history of experiencing anxiety, which has hampered her ability to work and function effectively in the past.

Grace has been working with Nicole for the past 4 months on developing more effective coping skills to reduce her anxiety. Nicole was initially standoffish and unhappy about being in the program or in therapy, but over time has grown to trust Grace. Nicole often comments that she appreciates Grace's help and that for the first time in her life she believes she is capable of succeeding. Because of the success in treatment and the positive working relationship that has developed, Grace often looks forward to meeting with Nicole. During one of their weekly sessions Nicole asks Grace if she has any children. Grace feels slightly uncomfortable and is unsure of how to respond, but to avoid making Nicole feel uncomfortable, shares that she does have children. During the following week's session, Nicole states that she would like to give Grace a children's book—one that she had collected for her children. She states that it was a favorite book of hers and that she would like for Grace to have it.

### Resolving the Ethical Dilemma

Think about the following questions. Write your answers down before moving on to the discussion.

1. What are the ethical dilemmas in this case?
2. Should Grace seek consultation?
3. Should she gather more information?
4. Based on a review of both the APA and ACA codes of ethics, which should Grace rely on to resolve this dilemma?
5. As you review the situation, do you think Grace should take the book from Nicole?

*(continued)*

## CASE STUDY VIGNETTE (continued)

Now that you have written down your answers, let us go together through what happened.

A good indicator of the presence of an ethical dilemma is the feeling of unease or confusion. In this case, treatment seemed to have been progressing well when the client presented a personal question to the counselor. These types of questions are common within therapy and have many motivations and functions within the therapeutic relationship. The client then informed the therapist that she would like to offer a gift. In this case, the therapist decided to share personal information but was later unsure of whether or not to receive a gift.

Regarding the issue of self-disclosure, it is necessary to consider the cultural and workplace norms regarding this type of personal disclosure, as well as whether personal disclosure is informed by the counselor's intrapsychic dynamics. The therapist, in this case, could have referred to either APA or ACA "Avoiding Harm" standards to determine the potential impact of this purposefully personal self-disclosure.

Regarding the issue of the gift, the therapist could have referred to APA Principle A, Do No Harm, or ACA Code A.10.f., Receiving Gifts, and considered the following variables: Nicole's cultural perception of giving and receiving gifts, how the gift-giving fits with or could affect the therapeutic relationship, the monetary value of the book, Nicole's motivation for giving the gift, and the counselor's motivation for wanting to accept or decline the gift.

### Case Study Discussion Questions

1. Which gray areas or slippery slopes were presented in this case?
2. Which actions within this vignette are important to note in order to best understand this situation?
3. To the individuals mentioned in this vignette, assign different sex, gender, sexual orientation, culture, socioeconomic status, nation of origin, immigrant status, refugee status, primary language spoken, disability, or other variables. Would any of these variables change your perception of the statements or actions within this vignette? If so, how? If not, what leads you to believe that none of these variables would impact your thinking or reactions? This information regarding your beliefs and reactions would be useful to discuss going forward in supervision.

## ACTIVITY 3.4

Discussing the feelings that we are having in reaction to our clients can be uncomfortable. Explore how you create conditions in which you would be comfortable enough to discuss your true reactions to your clients and your work. Which conditions would make this difficult? Can you create a situation with your peers in which they would be comfortable sharing their personal reactions with you?

# CHAPTER DISCUSSION QUESTIONS

1. What are some steps that I could follow in order to determine what is the "right" thing to do?
2. What are some blind spots that I may have regarding boundaries?
3. What kind of information can we ascertain from our wish to cross a boundary or a client's attempt at crossing a boundary?
4. Are there right and wrong actions? How can we tell what is truly "wrong" from what may be a gray area?

# CONCLUSION

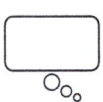

As was covered in this chapter, professional boundaries are maintained through an awareness of the cultural and workplace norms, and internal dynamics that impact a counselor's perception and experience of boundaries. Because boundaries may be crossed at times without being violated, it is important to acknowledge the contextual factors that are motivating the counselor's actions, as well as the impact upon the client.

## PERSONAL INVENTORY: QUESTIONS FOR FUTHER EXPLORATION

## PROFESSIONAL EXPERIENCES

1. Have you had an experience in the past in which your boss, manager, or professional superior seemed to step outside of their role when interacting with you? Can you recall what you were thinking or feeling in response to that? Can you recall how his or her actions may have affected your working relationship?
2. Have you had an experience at work or school in which you were friends with a coworker/fellow student? Can you recall how this impacted your work or school experience? Can you identify potential pros and cons of this relationship?

## PERSONAL EXPERIENCES

1. If you have been in therapy in the past, can you recall how the therapist maintained or did not maintain different types of boundaries? If so, can you recall your reaction to this as well as how this affected your working relationship?
2. Do you remember a time in the past when you went beyond your role to assist another person? Can you recall what prompted you to do so, how it turned out, and how you felt about it?

## FURTHER LEARNING AND SUGGESTED READING

Pope, K., & Keith-Spiegel, P. (2008). A practical approach to boundaries in psychotherapy: Making decisions, bypassing blunders, and mending fences. *Journal of Clinical Psychology: In Session, 64*(5), 638–652. doi:10.1002/jclp.20477

## REFERENCES

American Counseling Association. (2014). *2014 ACA code of ethics*. Retrieved from https://www.counseling.org/resources/aca-code-of-ethics.pdf

American Psychological Association. (2017). *Ethical principles of psychologists and code of conduct* (2002, amended June 1, 2010 and January 1, 2017). Retrieved from http://www.apa.org/ethics/code/index.aspx

Anderson, N. (2011). *Report of the Ethics Committee, 2010. American Psychologist, 66*(5), 393–403. doi:10.1037/a0024003

Beaulieu, C. (2004). Intercultural study of personal space: A case study. *Journal of Applied Social Psychology, 34*(4), 794–805. doi:10.1111/j.1559-1816.2004.tb02571

Celenza, A. (2007). *Sexual boundary violations: Therapeutic, supervisory, and academic contexts*. Lanham, MD: Jason Aronson.

Derlega, V., & Chaikin, A. (1977). Privacy and self-disclosure in social relationships. *Journal of Social Issues, 33*(3), 102–115. doi:10.1111/j.1540-4560.1977.tb01885

Fasasi, M. I., & Olowu, A. A. (2013). Boundary transgressions: An issue in psychotherapeutic encounter. *Ife Psychologia, 21*(3), 139–151.

Kozlowski, J., Pruitt, N., Dewalt, T., & Knox, S. (2014). Can boundary crossings in clinical supervision be beneficial? *Counselling Psychology Quarterly*, 1–18. doi:10.1080/09515070.2013.870123

Pope, K., Sonne, J., & Greene, B. (2006). *What therapists don't talk about and why: Understanding taboos that hurt us and our clients*. Washington, DC: American Psychological Association.

Pope, K., & Vetter, V. (1992). Ethical dilemmas encountered by members of the American Psychological Association. *American Psychologist, 47*, 397–411. doi:10.1037/0003-066X.47.3.397

Simone, D., McCarthy, P., & Skay, C. (1998). An investigation of client and counselor variables that influence likelihood of counselor self-disclosure. *Journal of Counseling & Development, 76*, 174–182. doi:10.1002/j.1556-6676.1998.tb02390

Zheng, P., Gray, M. J., Zhu, W.-Z., & Jiang, G.-R. (2014). Influence of culture on ethical decision making in psychology. *Ethics and Behavior, 24*, 510–522. doi:10.1080/10508422.2014.891075

# CHAPTER 4

# PROFESSIONAL COMPETENCE

*Professional competence* refers to our ability to perform effectively within our professional role. As counselors, we are required to remain aware of our professional strengths and weaknesses and respond accordingly when counseling situations fall outside of our ability to be effective. Professional competence involves working with client populations for which we have been properly trained, maintaining training and education throughout our careers, and identifying and addressing personal experiences or internal problems that can affect our ability to be effective counselors.

Specialty areas, such as forensic psychology and neuropsychology, have set procedures for developing and demonstrating competence. These are then used to acquire credentials as a forensic psychologist or a neuropsychologist. In order to gain this competence, one must acquire additional specialized training and receive supervision; at times, one may also take an additional exam. Counselors who do not go on to become formally specialized may still develop a specialty, or an area in which they spend an increased amount of time studying and practicing. Many counselors specialize in areas such as trauma or substance abuse. Although there may not be formal titles that indicate a counselor's ability to treat these specific issues, the expectation is that the counselor has engaged in learning, training, and additional practice for treatment of these specific issues.

Regardless of formal specialty or interest, all counselors are required to maintain their education throughout their career. Many counselors focus their continuing education within their specialty area, whereas others add clinical knowledge or practical knowledge on issues such as ethics or state laws. Not all state licensing boards require submission or proof of continuing education credits; some do so regularly and others do randomly every several years. Irrespective of state or licensing requirements, all counselors must maintain competence in the areas in which they practice through state-approved courses.

Maintaining professional competence through continuing education is a straightforward and easily attainable goal. Although upholding and improving your knowledge base throughout your career is important, equally significant to your functioning as a counselor is the recognition of areas where competence is lacking or compromised. Within this area, there are three common dilemmas: (a) having a general lack of experience during training and being asked to meet with a client with whom you have no experience, (b) recognizing and responding appropriately when a current client has issues for which you have not been trained, and (c) recognizing and responding appropriately when experiencing **personal problems** that may affect your work.

In this chapter, we cover what it means to be professionally competent, how to recognize when we are exceeding boundaries of competence, and how to maintain competence throughout a professional career. Professional competence includes a host of complex situations and variables. Much of the research and writings on the topic of competence focuses on multicultural competence (see Chapter 5). Understanding individual differences in our client population is essential for maintaining professional competence (Fisher, 2003).

### ACTIVITY 4.1

In Chapter 1, we reviewed the importance of self-awareness in arriving at sound ethical decisions. Return to Activity 1.4 and try to answer those questions as they relate to how your individual differences may impact your interpretation or reaction to the ethical dilemmas presented here. For example, are you aware of how your social identities that have socially constructed power (e.g., White, heterosexual, affluent, native English speaker) may impact your level of competence to work with clients who are different from you?

## HAVING A GENERAL UNDERSTANDING VERSUS HAVING THE NECESSARY TRAINING AND SKILLS

As time progresses, many counselors develop an approach toward treatment that is grounded in theory and guided by their experience. This approach may be applied to most of the counselor's clientele, regardless of the presenting problem, because the counselor has come to understand a person's condition through his or her theoretical framework. For example, a counselor may utilize the theory and practice of cognitive behaviorism, through which she is able to conceptualize a variety of issues or symptoms. This counselor, although able to conceptualize the causes and maintaining factors of a person's dysfunction, may not have training or experience directly related to the client's individual life experience. In other words, a counselor's ability to understand a person's issues does not necessarily indicate that counselor's ability or level of competence to treat a particular client.

As counselors develop throughout their careers, they also acquire a general knowledge base or understanding of most disorders or conditions. A **general understanding** includes knowledge regarding the causes, maintaining factors, and treatment approaches for a particular disorder or condition. For example, most counselors may have general knowledge about clients diagnosed with borderline personality disorder, such as the high incidence of histories of trauma, factors related to labile mood and behavior, and the empirically based dialectical behavioral therapy (DBT). However, a counselor may not have been trained in DBT, nor received training specific to this population. Given the potential severity of symptoms associated with some instances of this disorder, and others, acknowledging limits of professional competence is necessary.

> **GENERAL UNDERSTANDING** - A counselor's general understanding of aspects relevant to a particular disorder or population absent additional or specialized education, training, experience, or supervision.
>
> **NECESSARY TRAINING AND SKILLS** - A counselor's competence to treat a particular condition, or work with a particular population, based on the accumulation of a sufficient amount of education, training, experience, and supervision.

## WHAT ARE THE NECESSARY TRAINING AND SKILLS?

Professional competence, along with therapeutic alliance, is a factor that has been shown to positively impact results with some clients (Weck, Richtberg, Jakob, Neng, & Hofling, 2015). Developing interpersonal or relational skills is as important as gaining technical skills through modality-specific training. Skills that underlie a counselor's relational skills, or responsiveness, can be enhanced through education and supervision. According to Hatcher (2015), "responsiveness can be understood as 'knowing what to do and when' to advance the therapeutic work" (p. 755). Training and experience may improve a counselor's relational skills or responsiveness. However, other factors also impact a counselor's competence regarding responsiveness, as well as technical skill. Furthermore, scholars note that the **necessary training and skills** are not achieved by years of practice alone. According to Mollen, Kelly, and Ridely (2011), who have critiqued aspects of current counseling training models, "even advanced training and years of experience appear not to correlate strongly with expertise" (p. 921).

Thus, it is important to recognize that although education and training can provide a strong starting point for developing competence and expertise, they are not sufficient without further development. For example, in a study of perceptions of competence, doctoral trainees felt competent "in a range of areas by the time they applied for internship," although the authors stated that important areas of competence (e.g., research, assessment, intervention) appeared to instead develop over the course of their graduate training (Kamen, Veilleux, Bangen, VanderVeen, & Klonoff, 2010, p. 227). Thus, *feeling* competent does not necessarily translate to *being* competent.

Possessing competence therefore depends on several factors, including but not limited to the counselor's education, specific supervised training and amount of time in practice, counselor personality and other personal factors, as well as the client factors such as the severity of symptoms or personality structure.

Regarding the severity of symptoms, consider this example: A person who is diagnosed with borderline personality disorder and has a recent history of self-harm and hospitalizations for suicidal thoughts presents for treatment. In this case, the counselor should be someone who has the necessary training and skill, as opposed to a general understanding of the disorder. In contrast, if a person diagnosed with borderline personality disorder presents to treatment reporting conflict within relationships and moderate labile mood without any history of self-harm, suicidality, or hospitalizations, then a counselor with general knowledge, who is also able to receive additional education or consultation, may be appropriate. In essence, in terms of professional competence, the appropriateness to treat depends on the situation.

## PRACTICALLY SPEAKING, WHAT DO WE DO IF WE ARE NOT THE APPROPRIATE PERSON?

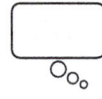

Whether clients are assigned, as is the case with trainees, or find treatment providers through independent practice, counselors hold the responsibility for identifying their level of competence to engage the client. Counselors are also responsible for determining if a client should be referred for more appropriate care. There are several practical ways to know if a counselor is the appropriate person to treat a particular client.

During emergency situations, meaning the counselor is the only available provider in that moment, there are guidelines regarding how to respond appropriately, even with limited training. The American Psychological Association's Code 2.02, Providing Services in Emergencies, states:

> *In emergencies, when psychologists provide services to individuals for whom other mental health services are not available and for which psychologists have not obtained the necessary training, psychologists may provide such services in order to ensure that services are not denied. The services are discontinued as soon as the emergency has ended or appropriate services are available. (American Psychological Association [APA], 2017, p. 5)*

The American Counseling Association (ACA) does not provide explicit direction regarding how to operate within emergency situations.

In instances where trainees are assigned a client by their supervisors, irrespective of their level of competence, the trainee must work cooperatively with his or her supervisor to determine if appropriate supervision, or other supports, will be enough to account for the lack of education, training, or experience on the part of the trainee. Both must remain aware of any limitations to the amount of supervision that is practically available given work or environmental constraints. For example, the workload of the supervisor may prevent him or her from providing the type of supervision the trainee needs (Schmidt, Ybanez-Llorente, & Lamb, 2013). Schmidt, Ybanez-Llorente, and Lamb noted:

> *Although SACs (substance abuse counselors) seem to desire supervision and seek guidance on legal and ethical issues from their supervisors, challenges facing supervisors in the addiction field, such as large caseloads, few resources, and limited training, may lessen the quality of supervision they provide. (p. 87)*

Counselors who work within a structure that includes a supervisor or director who helps to manage the client assignment may need to make their own determination that they are not competent to treat a client, and must then ask that they be reassigned. Although there may be pressures to avoid reassignments based on work dynamics or the work structure, counselors themselves are responsible for these types of decisions. Conversely, supervisors may point out when a trainee or counselor needs to refer a client to another provider due to a lack of competence. The presence of a supervisor provides important insight into the level of competence, particularly when the supervisor is closely involved in the counselor's actions through case reviews, education, and process-oriented supervision. In these instances, although the supervisor's involvement may generate reactions, it is important for counselors to be receptive, acknowledge the reality that "we don't know what we don't know," and respond accordingly.

Lastly, counselors must have readily available names and numbers for alternative treatment providers should a referral become necessary. For example, consider a client who arrives for an initial session reporting that she has been diagnosed with anorexia nervosa and is looking for treatment for this eating disorder. If a counselor does not have the necessary training and skills to work effectively with this client, he or she must identify referral sources with the necessary training and skills. This may require some research on the part of the counselor to determine the appropriate referral. Counselors must be prepared to provide relevant referrals.

Multiple variables must be considered when determining if one is professionally competent to treat a particular individual or engage in a particular clinical task. The weight of each variable, such as education, training, experience, and client variables, depends on the situation. If one is not the appropriate counselor, a referral must be made to an appropriate and competent provider. How the referral is enacted depends on the treatment environment and the needs of the client. In short, the decision to treat or refer is guided by our responsibility to identify whether our abilities match the client's need.

Among the many gray areas that pose ethical dilemmas are three that we review in this chapter: (a) being assigned a client who is experiencing symptoms or a situation for which the counselor has not been specially trained (a common dilemma, especially for counselors early in their careers); (b) awareness of a personal problem that may be affecting one's work; and (c) maintaining professional competence.

## ACTIVITY 4.2

Can you remember the last time you were asked to complete a task but you knew that you were not properly prepared or capable? Reflect on the circumstances and attempt to recall your reactions as well as your thought process that allowed you to recognize that you were not the right person to complete this task.

# SELF-ASSESSMENT: CURRENT BELIEFS AND EXPECTATIONS

## Instructions

If you were to take an essay test, how well would you be able to answer the following questions critically and thoroughly? Give yourself a letter grade from A to F. Be honest. There are no right or wrong answers when learning where you stand.

## Beliefs Regarding Professional Competence

- Role of the Counselor
  - What do you think is the role of a counselor in maintaining professional competence? Think of what your role does and does not consist of, as well as what you believe your responsibilities are.
  - What is the responsibility of the counselor regarding the maintenance of his or her own mental health and well-being?
  - What is the responsibility of a counselor in maintaining competence after it is initially gained?
- Role of the Client
  - What is the responsibility of a client in providing information necessary for you to determine if you are the appropriate provider to treat that client?
  - What are your expectations of how much information clients should share about themselves during the initial phone call or initial sessions?
- Function of Competence
  - What may be some benefits of developing and maintaining professional competence?
  - Do you think that there are some issues with which you might be able to develop some competence while in the midst of treating a client?
  - What personal factors may impede your ability to perform effectively as a clinician?

Think of cultural variables or situational variables that may impact your ability to maintain professional competence.

## Expectations

- Successes in Treatment
  - What do you think is the role of professional competence in the success of treatment?

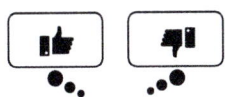

- Situations That May Be Challenging
  - In general, which types of situations or environments would create challenges for maintaining your competence as a therapist?
  - In general, which situational variables may impact your ability to recognize your level of competence?
- Situations That May Create Ethical Dilemmas
  - What are two situations that would *likely* create an ethical dilemma for you when dealing with issues related to competence?
  - Think of yourself specifically: What is it about your experience with competence and incompetence that would likely impact your thinking and behavior within the context of treatment?
- Methods for Maintaining Competence
  - What do you actually do to maintain competence? Think of immediate and ongoing actions as well as inner processes.

# ETHICAL STANDARDS SURROUNDING PROFESSIONAL COMPETENCE

First, it is important to understand where one can read about professional competence in both codes of ethics. Both the American Psychological Association (APA, 2017) and the American Counseling Association (ACA, 2014) approach the issue of professional competence similarly, focusing on the effectiveness of the counselor and standards for maintaining his or her effectiveness. Depending on the ethical issue you are trying to resolve, you may find references to professional competence in multiple areas in the code of ethics. Therefore, it is always important to untangle the dilemma and recognize the need to refer to multiple codes, as well as the principles.

## APA Ethical Principles of Psychologists and Code of Conduct

The APA Ethical Principles of Psychologists and Code of Conduct includes a section designated for "competence." This section describes competence as well as the standards for maintaining competence. Although other principles can drive our understanding of competence, Principle D: Justice provides direction that is directly relevant to this standard. It states:

> *Psychologists recognize that fairness and justice entitle all persons to access to and benefit from the contributions of psychology and to equal quality in the processes, procedures, and services being conducted by psychologists. Psychologists exercise reasonable judgment and take precautions to ensure that their potential biases, the boundaries of their competence, and the limitations of their expertise do not lead to or condone unjust practices.* (APA, 2017, p. 4)

## ACA Code of Ethics

The ACA Code of Ethics also addresses obligations regarding professional competence in multiple sections, including an inspirational introduction in Section C: Professional Responsibility:

> Counselors aspire to open, honest, and accurate communication in dealing with the public and other professionals. Counselors facilitate access to counseling services, and they practice in a nondiscriminatory manner within the boundaries of professional and personal competence; they also have a responsibility to abide by the ACA Code of Ethics. . . . (ACA, 2014, p. 8)

# DIFFERENCES AND OVERLAP

In this chapter, we focus on three ethical dilemmas summarized in the following practical questions: (a) Am I the appropriate counselor for this person? (b) Is my personal situation affecting my work? (c) How do I maintain professional competence? We review each of these dilemmas and walk through how both APA and ACA can guide our ethical decisions.

## Dilemma 1: Am I the Appropriate Counselor for This Person?

Although identifying the level of competence to treat a particular client may seem to be a straightforward task, several variables may impact our ability to effectively make this assessment.

Some evidence has shown that less experienced or "newly qualified" psychologists tend to rate themselves higher on competencies when compared with more experienced psychologists (Kuittinen, Merilainen, & Raty, 2014). When early professionals lack experience, they may also lack the sufficient capacity to recognize limitations. According to Dunning, Johnson, Ehrlinger, and Kruger (2003), individuals' perceived competence is often measured by ideas about skill level. Therefore, judgment is based on a subjective evaluation, rather than on objective measure, of achievement. Conversely, many counselors-in-training question their competence, especially in response to negative reactions from their clients (Goodman, 2005).

At times, lack of congruency between perceived and actual competence can be explained by a counselor's motivations to work with a particular population or treat a specific client. For example, there may be internal motivations for wanting to treat a client of which the counselor is not immediately aware. Given a client's motivation to view the counselor as competent or as someone who can help, counselors may also struggle to manage their reactions to a client's perception and fail to recognize their lack of competence. There are also times when counselors may be eager to treat a client in order to impress their supervisors, or as a way to be helpful so that a case need not be reassigned. In private practice settings, the motivation may be monetary. These motivations could impede a counselor's ability to recognize the need for a consultation or possible referral.

Both the APA and ACA ethical codes provide direction regarding personal assessment of competence. Counselors can determine their appropriateness to treat a specific client by referring to ethical standards regarding boundaries of competence in the APA and ACA codes. Both sets of standards are consistent in their descriptions of professional competence.

*APA Code 2.01, Boundaries of Competence: (a) Psychologists provide services, teach, and conduct research with populations and in areas only within the boundaries of their competence, based on their education, training, supervised experience, consultation, study, or professional experience. (b) Where scientific or professional knowledge in the discipline of psychology establishes that an understanding of factors associated with age, gender, gender identity, race, ethnicity, culture, national origin, religion, sexual orientation, disability, language, or socioeconomic status is essential for effective implementation of their services or research, psychologists have or obtain the training, experience, consultation, or supervision necessary to ensure the competence of their services, or they make appropriate referrals, except as provided in Standard 2.02, Providing Services in Emergencies. (APA, 2017, p. 5)*

*ACA Code C.2.a., Boundaries of Competence: Counselors practice only within the boundaries of their competence, based on their education, training, supervised experience, state and national professional credentials, and appropriate professional experience. Whereas multicultural counseling competency is required across all counseling specialties, counselors gain knowledge, personal awareness, sensitivity, dispositions, and skills pertinent to being a culturally competent counselor in working with a diverse client population. (ACA, 2014, p. 8)*

Notice that both set of standards require appropriate training and knowledge, as well as the importance of having multicultural competence (see Chapter 5).

When taking on new clients, many counselors create an initial screening process to determine if they are the appropriate person to provide treatment. A common method is to ask the client the reason for which he or she is seeking treatment, along with information regarding the client's psychiatric history, and past and current functioning. One purpose of this screening is to ascertain whether a referral to another source is immediately needed prior to entering into a therapeutic relationship.

Once a client has been accepted for treatment, counselors are tasked with regularly determining if they remain appropriate or competent. For example, a counselor who is trained in, and comfortable with, treating depression may take on a client who is experiencing depression. However, during the course of treatment, this client may begin to decline and experience regular suicidality. At this point, the counselor is tasked with determining if he or she is competent to provide the necessary treatment given the treatment method, and the counselor's training and knowledge of other resources. Variables such as whether the counselor has an on-call service for emergencies, is familiar with inpatient or other services that could be required if an emergency arises, has a history of working specifically with clients who are actively suicidal, and has training in effectively assessing for suicidality should all be considered. Whereas a counselor could initially be competent to treat a client, an issue may present itself that would subsequently result in the need for a referral to a more appropriate counselor or treatment provider.

One method for determining if clients should initially be accepted or referred is to determine if their presenting problems could be best treated by a specialist, another treatment method, or just another more knowledgeable treatment provider. Examples of specialty areas include, but are not limited to, substance abuse, trauma, pain management, developmental disorders, certain personality disorders, and domestic violence. If a counselor is not specifically knowledgeable and trained in specialty areas, then a referral may be appropriate. An alternative to a referral may be to recommend an additional treatment source, such as a therapy group, if there is another presenting problem for which the counselor is an appropriate treatment provider. For example, if a counselor is competent to treat social phobia but the client also has a history of trauma, given the severity of the symptoms related to the trauma, recommending a trauma support group in addition to the counselor's treatment of the social phobia may be appropriate. Consultation is always a useful source for making these determinations.

Regarding the treatment method, some clients may be best served by group therapy, or by a higher level of care, such as a partial or intensive outpatient program. Depending on the severity of symptoms and level of functioning, a counselor must determine if the treatment modality is appropriate given the client's needs.

Finally, there may be populations for which a counselor is not competent without training on the role of culture or context. Examples of such populations may include, but are not limited to, veterans; people who are incarcerated or were formerly incarcerated; immigrant groups; those who are undocumented; refugees; people of color; lesbian, gay, bisexual, transgender, and queer (LGBTQ) individuals; older adults; children; or parents. As noted earlier, APA Code 2.01b, Boundaries of Competence, requires that the counselor have the training, experience, and consultation needed to provide culturally competent treatment (APA, 2017). Similarly, the ACA Code of Ethics, C.2.a., Boundaries of Competence, also noted previously, requires cultural competence irrespective of specialty (ACA, 2014).

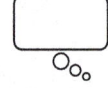

Gaining the necessary skills to acquire cultural competence can be accomplished through education, training, and supervision. It is important to mention that history of exposure to, or even counseling with, a particular population does not necessarily create cultural competence. In addition to the requirements mentioned in boundaries of competence codes, ACA Code E.5.b., Cultural Sensitivity, provides clarification around competence.

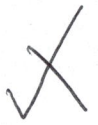

*Counselors recognize that culture affects the manner in which clients' problems are defined and experienced. Clients' socioeconomic and cultural experiences are considered when diagnosing mental disorders. (ACA, 2014, p. 11)*

Similarly, APA includes direct mention of these issues through Principle E: Respect for People's Rights and Dignity, which states:

*Psychologists respect the dignity and worth of all people, and the rights of individuals to privacy, confidentiality, and self-determination. Psychologists are aware that special safeguards may be necessary to protect the rights and welfare of persons or communities whose vulnerabilities impair autonomous decision making. Psychologists are aware of and respect cultural, individual, and role differences, including those based on age, gender, gender identity, race, ethnicity, culture, national origin, religion, sexual orientation, disability, language, and socioeconomic status, and consider these factors when working with members of such groups. Psychologists try to eliminate the effect on their work of biases based on those factors, and they do not knowingly participate in or condone activities of others based upon such prejudices. (APA, 2017, p. 4)*

Specific training and supervision can assist counselors in becoming aware of their own biases and assumptions, as well as areas of privilege that often present a blind spot (see Chapter 8). The importance of self-awareness is further underscored by APA's "Guidelines on Multicultural Education, Training, Research, Practice, and Organizational Change for Psychologists." Included in the guidelines are the following:

*Guideline 1: Psychologists are encouraged to recognize that, as cultural beings, they may hold attitudes and beliefs that can detrimentally influence their perceptions of and interactions with individuals who are ethnically and racially different from themselves. (APA, 2002, p. 382)*

*Guideline 2: Psychologists are encouraged to recognize the importance of multicultural sensitivity/responsiveness to, knowledge of, and understanding about ethnically and racially different individuals. (APA, 2002, p. 385)*

## How Do We Make Referrals?

Counselors are responsible for identifying the changing needs of their clients or situations that may warrant a referral. Initial screenings are useful because they allow counselors to offer referrals prior to building a connection with the client. At that point, a counselor should research and provide specific referral options for care. However, if a referral becomes necessary at any point during treatment, the counselor should be sensitive to the experience of the client who is now being referred to another professional. Although the goal is to provide the best possible care for the client, the client may experience a variety of reactions to the referral. One method for maintaining the integrity of the relationship is to provide the client with clear reasons for the need for the referral and to suggest working together to gather potential referral sources. Despite the reality that referring a client may cause discomfort in both counselor and client, it is the counselor's responsibility to identify the boundaries of his or her competence and recognize when a client will be best served by another professional.

## ACTIVITY 4.3

Given the reports that new clinicians overestimate their competence when compared with more experienced clinicians, let's try a self-reflection exercise.

Think of your most recent experience with gaining an additional skill or understanding with a particular diagnosis or population.

1. Identify your areas of competence with regard to this diagnosis or population. (Be as specific as possible. List all of your education and training related to the areas that create your competency.)

2. Now, rate your competency with the skills you just listed on a scale from 1 to 10, with 1 being not competent to treat and 10 being the most qualified person to treat.

3. Go back now and fill out all of the numbers around your self-score. For example, if you scored yourself as having a competency rating of 6, identify why and then identify what a 5 or 7 level of competency would entail. For example, identify what would make you slightly more or slightly less competent.

4. Articulate why your score is sufficient to treat this population, and indicate what variables could come into play that would reduce your score. Work with those around you on this step in order to reduce any blind spots. For example, encourage others around you to express feedback regarding your perceived competence, as well as any cultural variables or experience that may impact your score.

## Dilemma 2: Is My Personal Situation Affecting My Work?

Recognizing the ways in which personal situations may be affecting our work can be a complicated task. Throughout our careers, there are many situations that can, and will, impact the quality of our mental health and our work. Although many counselors attempt to prevent their "home life" from affecting their "work life," a true separation between home and work is somewhat difficult to accomplish. Life events such as financial difficulties, health problems, family issues, or personal conflicts will likely happen at varying points which can impact a counselor's well-being.

In addition to personal situations, work environments may also impact a counselor's functioning given the type and amount of stressors. Examples of work environments that can create stress and affect personal health include, but are not limited to, inpatient hospitals, correctional environments, isolated work situations, and overburdened community mental health agencies. In addition to personal situations and work environments, working with certain client populations may lead to personal stress. For example, working with clients who have experienced extreme trauma, those who are violent, or those who are frequently suicidal can take a toll on the counselor's mental health (see Chapter 8).

We can refer to specific APA and ACA ethical codes to understand the importance of recognizing if our personal situations are affecting our work.

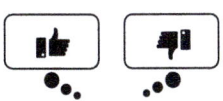

> *APA Code 2.06, Personal Problems and Conflicts: (a) Psychologists refrain from initiating an activity when they know or should know that there is a substantial likelihood that their personal problems will prevent them from performing their work-related activities in a competent manner. (b) When psychologists become aware of personal problems that may interfere with their performing work-related duties adequately, they take appropriate measures, such as obtaining professional consultation or assistance, and determine whether they should limit, suspend, or terminate their work-related duties. (See also Standard 10.10, Terminating Therapy) (APA, 2017, p. 5)*

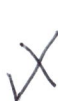

> *ACA Code F.5.b., Impairment: Students and supervisees monitor themselves for signs of **impairment** from their own physical, mental, or emotional problems and refrain from offering or providing professional services when such impairment is likely to harm a client or others. They notify their faculty and/or supervisors and seek assistance for problems that reach the level of professional impairment, and, if necessary, they limit, suspend, or terminate their professional responsibilities until it is determined that they may safely resume their work. (ACA, 2014, p. 13)*

Personal well-being impacts the quality of the services provided to clients. This includes the ability to be objective, attentive, self-aware or mindful of personal reactions, patient, flexible, and motivated. Counselors are responsible for regularly monitoring their functioning and effectiveness. Some counselors rely on how they feel, such as recognizing when they are feeling consistently tired, frustrated, avoidant, or uninterested in providing services. Other counselors attempt to use behavioral markers to identify whether their work is being affected, such as noticing if they are forgetting appointments or details, experiencing changes in daily routines, or noticing that they are ruminating about specific clients outside of work.

Recognizing that experiencing any kind of stress does not necessarily affect our competence, how can we tell when it is? The best way is to seek consultation or supervision. Understanding that we can all lack the ability to be objective, especially while experiencing a significant personal difficulty or stress, the best method is to ask for assistance. Counselors can check with fellow workplace colleagues to see if they notice changes or have concerns. Supervision can also be beneficial, as can consultation with a professional who is familiar with the counselor's typical functioning and willing to provide objective feedback. If personal issues are impacting the ability to offer competent services, counselors must provide a referral in the most appropriate manner possible.

When counselors experience personal problems, but not to the extent that these impact counseling practice, they can take steps to preserve their competence and maintain the quality of their work despite the personal difficulties (see Chapter 8).

> **IMPAIRMENT** - Conditions under which a counselor is no longer able to be effective or appropriate as a result of internal variables that have affected her or his professional functioning.

## Dilemma 3: How Do I Maintain My Professional Competence?

Many counselors begin with a particular area of interest that guides their choice in work or training sites. From this point forward, counselors have begun to build their knowledge base and professional experience. Throughout our careers, many of us develop specialties or areas of interest that guide our choice in client population or type of work. As mentioned previously, to gain our initial competence level, we must have experienced a sufficient amount of education, training, and supervision to treat specific populations. Once this competence is gained, counselors are responsible for maintaining this competence through their careers, or as long as they continue with that specific type of work or with that specific client population.

To understand how to maintain this competence, we can look to both the APA and ACA ethical codes.

> APA Code 2.03, *Maintaining Competence*: Psychologists undertake ongoing efforts to develop and maintain their competence. (APA, 2017, p. 5)

> ACA Code C.2.f., *Continuing Education*: Counselors recognize the need for continuing education to acquire and maintain a reasonable level of awareness of current scientific and professional information in their fields of activity. Counselors maintain their competence in the skills they use, are open to new procedures, and remain informed regarding best practices for working with diverse populations. (ACA, 2014, p. 9)

Many states require a yearly accumulation of continuing education credits to maintain a professional license. Workshops and trainings offered by state associations, educational institutions, or by private treatment providers apply for and are granted the ability to award continuing education credits to those who attend their workshop or training. These are often valuable opportunities to connect with treatment providers around a specific treatment issue. Regardless of the need for credits to maintain a professional license, there is a need to maintain up-to-date information and skills based on the latest evidence-based techniques and data. What the counselor knows today will likely change, or at least be modified, over time given its application to a variety of populations.

### CASE STUDY VIGNETTE

#### Instructions

Following the case study vignette, we will walk through some questions on how to make an ethical decision to resolve this dilemma. Remember to monitor your reactions, keeping track of any that include shaming the counselor for "bad" behavior or for being a "bad counselor." Focus on the internal and external factors that may have led to this behavior. Now is

*(continued)*

## CASE STUDY VIGNETTE (continued)

the time to notice if there are any patterns in your reactions, or the substance of your reactions, and to discuss these in supervision and consultation. This is valuable information for your reflection on what some of your personal biases and blind spots may be. (See the Appendix, Typical Cognitive and Emotional Reactions, at the end of this book.)

### Case Study

*Althea is working at a community mental health center where she provides individual therapy. She earned her hours for licensure here and was recently hired to work full time. The expectation is that each clinician will maintain 30 clients on his or her caseload; clients are assigned randomly and according to the clinician's openings.*

*Althea has been working weekly with James, a 36-year-old White male veteran, for the past 3 months. When therapy began, he asked for help with anxiety and his relationship with his wife. He currently lives with his wife and two children but has been out of work for the past 2 years due to his symptoms. Althea began to provide assistance with anxiety-reducing techniques as well as communication strategies for James and his wife. James reported that this was helpful, resulting in a slight reduction in anxiety but no change in his relationship with his wife. Althea feels comfortable with and motivated to help James. Although she has not shared this with James, she feels motivated and interested to help because her spouse is also a veteran and has experienced similar issues.*

*Last week James revealed that he has been binging and purging on a daily basis; he explained that he has done so "on and off" for the past 15 years. He indicated that he is not aware of the motivations for his behavior. He denied ever having help with this, stating that he has been embarrassed to talk about it up until now. He shared that he now feels comfortable with Althea and is open to finally receiving help. He also revealed an extensive history of trauma, including sexual abuse as a child by his stepfather as well as two deployments to Iraq that lasted 1 year each.*

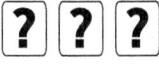

*Althea acknowledges that she has not had specific training for eating disorders and has not had any specific training in treating trauma outside of what she received through two classes during her graduate program. She is aware that she has built a positive working relationship with James and now feels responsible to continue with him given his statements regarding his comfort with and hope to receive help from her.*

### Resolving the Ethical Dilemma

Think about the following questions. Write your answers down before moving on to the discussion.

1. What are the ethical dilemmas in this case?
2. Should Althea stop to seek consultation?
3. Should Althea gather more information? Which information should she gather?

*(continued)*

## CASE STUDY VIGNETTE (continued)

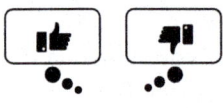

4. Based on the review of the APA and ACA codes of ethics, which should be relied on to resolve this dilemma?
5. As you review the situation, should Althea continue to treat James?
6. Are there any issues that are affecting Althea's competence to effectively treat James?

Now that you have written down your answers, let us go together through what happened.

We now know that a good indicator of the presence of an ethical dilemma is a feeling of unease or confusion. In this case, treatment seemed to be progressing adequately when the client shared additional information regarding his symptoms with the therapist. These types of occurrences are common within therapy and present the need to be thoughtful regarding what is appropriate as well as what is possible (which options are actually available). In this case, the therapist feels conflicted because of her responsibility to the client to maintain the working relationship as well as the responsibility to be able to provide the appropriate care given her lack of training.

Regarding the ethical issues present in this vignette, the most significant dilemma is whether Althea should continue to treat James given her apparent lack of knowledge and experience regarding some of his prominent issues. Althea does not possess the necessary skills for effectively treating an eating disorder, nor issues related to trauma. Given the severity of James's symptoms (he has been out of work for 2 years), it would be appropriate to consider alternative forms of care. One option would be to work with James to find a different treatment provider who specializes in eating disorders or the specific types of trauma that James has experienced. An alternative solution may be for James to attend additional therapy through groups or some other method while Althea continues to work with him within her competence, which is to treat his anxiety. If James's anxiety has resolved and he is now only experiencing symptoms of his eating disorder and issues related to child abuse and trauma from his military experience, then it is time for this counselor to refer him to a new counselor who can appropriately meet his needs. Refer to the following codes for further exploration: APA's (2017) standards 2.01(a) and (b), Boundaries of Competence, and 10.10, Terminating Therapy; ACA's (2014) standards C.2.a., Boundaries of Competence, and A.11., Termination and Referral.

### Case Study Discussion Questions

1. Which variables within this vignette are important to note to best understand this situation?
2. Which information is left out or should be clarified to better understand the nature of this dilemma?

*(continued)*

## CASE STUDY VIGNETTE (continued)

3. What type of education, training, or supervision would have increased this therapist's competence to the point that she could be effective?
4. What may have been an appropriate and respectful approach to discussing the referral with James? What may have been James's reaction when informed that he would be referred to another professional?
5. You may have noticed the comment that the counselor's husband was also a veteran. What steps could this counselor have taken to monitor her effectiveness or objectivity given her personal connection to some of her client's issues?
6. What recommendations would you make to increase the level of competence around issues related to eating disorders, trauma, or the veteran population?

# CHAPTER DISCUSSION QUESTIONS

1. What are some practical methods for gaining and maintaining competence in your area of work, given your career stage? Can you identify local organizations that provide further trainings and workshops? Can you identify state or national guidelines for determining your competence to practice in this area, or to refer to yourself as a specialist? Work with your colleagues to investigate how to increase your competencies. Even better, make plans with some of your colleagues to attend an educational workshop within your area of interest.
2. What methods do you use to recognize areas or situations that may exceed your level of competence?
3. What methods do you use to monitor your effectiveness? What ways can you engage supervision and consultation toward this effort?
4. Are you interested in a particular specialty area?

# CONCLUSION

Professional competence depends on the accurate acknowledgment of our skills or ability within a certain area, the ability to identify when personal problems are negatively affecting our functioning, and dedication to maintaining competency throughout our career. Maintaining competence requires ongoing self-reflection and openness to acknowledge limitations to better serve our clients.

## PERSONAL INVENTORY: QUESTIONS FOR FUTHER EXPLORATION

### PROFESSIONAL EXPERIENCES

1. Have you had an experience in the past in which an authority figure seemed to lack the competence to be able to properly understand or help you? Can you recall what you were thinking or feeling in response to that? Can you recall how those thoughts and feelings may have impacted your working relationship or your behavior?

2. Have you had an experience at work or school in which you became aware that you lacked the ability to complete a particular task? Can you recall your reaction to this as well as the steps you took to proceed? Looking back, are there other steps you could have taken?

### PERSONAL EXPERIENCES

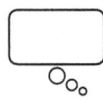

1. Can you remember the last time that a personal problem affected your work? How could you tell? Can you recall cognitive, emotional, and behavioral indicators that your work was being affected?

2. Can you think of cultural factors or other variables related to your background that would impact your ability or motivation to acknowledge when you are not prepared or professionally competent? What steps could you take to increase the likelihood that you would be open to acknowledging when you are in need of more support or training?

## REFERENCES

American Counseling Association. (2014). *2014 ACA code of ethics.* Retrieved from https://www.counseling.org/resources/aca-code-of-ethics.pdf

American Psychological Association. (2002). Guidelines on multicultural education, training, research, practice, and organizational change for psychologists. *American Psychologist, 58*(5), 377–402. doi:10.1037/0003-066X.58.5.377

American Psychological Association. (2017). *Ethical principles of psychologists and code of conduct* (2002, amended June 1, 2010 and January 1, 2017). Retrieved from http://www.apa.org/ethics/code/index.aspx

Dunning, D., Johnson, K., Ehrlinger, J., & Kruger, J. (2003). Why people fail to recognize their own incompetence. *Current Directions in Psychological Science, 12,* 83–87. doi:10.1111/1467-8721.01235

Fisher, C. (2003). *Decoding the ethics code: A practical guide for psychologists.* Thousand Oaks, CA: Sage.

Goodman, G. (2005). I feel stupid and contagious: Countertransference reactions of fledgling clinicians to patients who have negative therapeutic reactions. *American Journal of Psychotherapy, 59,* 149–168.

Hatcher, R. (2015). Interpersonal competencies: Responsiveness, technique, and training in psychotherapy. *American Psychologist, 70,* 747–757. doi:10.1037/a0039803

Kamen, C., Veilleux, J., Bangen, K., VanderVeen, J., & Klonoff, E. (2010). Climbing the stairway to competency: Trainee perspectives on competency development. *Training and Education in Professional Psychology, 4,* 227–234. doi:10.1037/a0021092

Kuittinen, M., Merilainen, M., & Raty, H. (2014). Professional competences of young psychologists: The dimensions of self-rated competence domains and their variation in early years of the psychologist's careers. *European Journal of Psychology of Education, 29*(1), 63–80. doi:10.1007/s10212-013-0187-0

Mollen, D., Kelly, S., & Ridely, C. (2011). Therapeutic change: The raison d'être for counseling competence. *The Counseling Psychologist, 36,* 918–927.

Schmidt, E. A., Ybanez-Llorente, K., & Lamb, B. (2013). Enhancing supervision in the addictions field: Introducing the supervisor evaluation of the professional and ethical competence of substance abuse counselors. *Alcoholism Treatment Quarterly, 31,* 1–18. doi:10.1080/07347324.2013.746624

Weck, F., Richtberg, S., Jakob, M., Neng, J., & Hofling, V. (2015). Therapist competence and therapeutic alliance are important in the treatment of health anxiety (hypochondriasis). *Psychiatry Research, 228,* 53–58. doi:10.1016/j.psychres.2015.03.042

# PART III DYNAMIC AND CONTEMPORARY ETHICAL ISSUES

# CHAPTER 5

# CULTURALLY COMPETENT TREATMENT

Over the past several decades, we have seen a surge in research, guidelines, and policies that underscore the importance of providing services that incorporate clients' worldviews and historical–political realities. However, research that examines disparities based on sociodemographic characteristics (e.g., age, gender, ethnic background) paints a somewhat gloomy picture. For example, it is well documented that most racial and ethnic minorities underutilize mainstream mental health services. The underutilization can be explained by a host of factors—from lack of access to treatment to language barriers. In addition, despite service need, once ethnic and racial minority clients seek mental health services, it is also documented that they receive poorer quality of services. Clients often experience the counselor as aloof, emotionally disconnected, or simply out of touch with the reality of their problems. In fact, when therapy is devoid of such contextual realities, research shows it accounts for poor treatment engagement, cultural mistrust, failed appointments, and premature termination (for reviews, see Arredondo, Gallardo-Cooper, Delgado-Romero, & Zapata, 2014; Mio, Barker, & Tumambing, 2016; Sue & Sue, 2013).

Therefore, counselors must ensure that all individuals, regardless of background or sociodemographic characteristics, receive adequate treatment—and one that is relevant to their specific sociodemographic realities. Accordingly, both the American Psychological Association (hereafter referred to as APA; APA, 2017) and the American Counseling Association (hereafter referred to as ACA; ACA, 2014) have dedicated guidelines. Most recently, the *Diagnostic and Statistical Manual of Mental Disorders* (*DSM-5*) also included a cultural formulation interview guide for counselors to assess the role of cultural, historical, and contextual factors in the mental health of clients (American Psychiatric Association, 2014).

## CULTURAL COMPETENCE

In Chapter 4, we reviewed the ethical codes and guidelines associated with professional competence. We did not, however, discuss issues specific to cultural competence, although these are outlined within the same codes. Because cultural competence is complex, we use this chapter to go into detail regarding its complexity.

In the seminal and often cited works by Arredondo and Sue (Arredondo et al., 1996; Sue et al., 1982; Sue, Arredondo, & McDavis, 1996), they offered a framework for the components needed to provide culturally competent treatment, or for being multiculturally competent as a counselor. This included the importance of self-awareness, knowledge, and skills.

## MULTICULTURAL COMPETENCE

1. *Awareness*: Counselors understand the beliefs, attitudes, and biases they hold toward marginalized populations.

2. *Knowledge*: Counselors acquire knowledge about their own worldview (i.e., based on their own racial, cultural, ethnic, social class, gender identities) and those of the populations they serve.

3. *Skills*: Counselors acquire the skills, strategies, and interventions that are relevant to diverse populations.

At face value, the components of competence appear quite straightforward. Training and education can inform our level of competence, to an extent, as it relates to knowledge of clients who may be different from ourselves. However, there is a shortage of culturally responsive research (Arredondo et al., 2014; Mazzula, 2015) to inform both theory and practice with diverse populations. Therefore, the extent to which counselors can gain the knowledge needed to deliver culturally competent treatment remains limited.

A host of complex nuances must be considered in culturally competent care. For example, when conducting psychological assessments, basic knowledge is needed to select appropriately normed and validated assessment tools for the client population. Screening tools must be available in the preferred language of the client. While this is basic knowledge, we argue that given the lack of culturally relevant research to inform practice, counselors may continue to use assessment tools that may not be relevant or appropriate with diverse populations. Beyond basic knowledge of norms and validity, there are nuances that require more in-depth attention—for example, cultural beliefs and values must be considered (Mazzula & Torres, 2017). Some cultural groups prefer to engage in personal relationships that are grounded in values of family, reciprocity, and friendliness. Clients who endorse these values may provide socially desirable responses to maintain a positive relationship with the counselor. One of the challenges to providing culturally competent treatment is that it requires knowledge of those being treated that is beyond what can be learned from basic courses or continuing education training. It also requires critical self-reflection of the counselor's personal life experiences and worldviews, and knowledge of how these inform the counselor's interactions, conceptualizations, and treatment approach.

# SELF-ASSESSMENT: CURRENT BELIEFS AND EXPECTATIONS

## Instructions

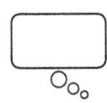

If you were to take an essay test, how well would you be able to answer the following questions critically and thoroughly? Give yourself a letter grade from A to F. Be honest. There are no right or wrong answers when learning where you stand.

## Beliefs

- Role of the Counselor
  - What is the role of a counselor in maintaining cultural competence?
- Role of the Client
  - What is the role of a client in knowing what values, beliefs, and assumptions impact his or her mental health?
  - What is the role of clients in teaching their counselor about issues of culture when the counselor is not from the same background?
- Function of Cultural Competence
  - What is the benefit of a counselor's cultural competence in the client–therapist relationship?
  - What may be a challenge in maintaining cultural competence in the client–therapist relationship?

## Expectations

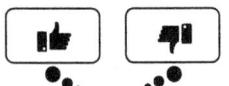

- Successes in Treatment
  - What is the role of cultural competence in the success of treatment?
- Situations That May Be Challenging
  - What are two situations in which it may be personally challenging for you to maintain cultural competence?
- Situations That May Create Ethical Dilemmas
  - What are two situations that would create an ethical dilemma for you when dealing with issues of multiculturalism?
- Methods for Maintaining Cultural Competence
  - What do you personally do to ensure that you are a culturally competent counselor?

- Impact on Self and Professional Growth
  - What is the role of cultural competence in your personal development as an individual and your professional growth as a counselor who is ever-evolving?

## SOCIAL–POLITICAL REALITIES

Before we discuss specific ethical standards regarding culturally competent treatment, we review critical issues and social-political realities that may impact how clients engage treatment, how they heal, and how they recover. Although going into detail with each aspect of this topic is beyond the scope of the book, we briefly review points that are necessary to consider. Be cautioned that there are significant within-group differences, which means that information regarding a group may not be applicable to all of its members. Further assessment will always be necessary to determine each client's specific needs, as well her or his unique sociodemographic characteristics and realities.

### Acculturation

*Acculturation* is an umbrella term used to describe changes in behavior, thoughts, and beliefs that result from encounters with a new host culture. Acculturation stressors may increase the risk for psychiatric disorders, such as depression and anxiety. For some immigrant groups, the longer they live in the United States, the higher the risk of mental health problems (Alegria et al., 2007; Arredondo et al., 2014; National Alliance on Mental Illness [NAMI], 2009). As individuals acculturate, their worldviews may change. For example, recent studies show that the rise in suicide attempts among Latina adolescent girls may be explained in part by familial conflicts related to worldviews. Therefore, proper assessment of the extent to which clients' acculturation experiences impact mental health is critical.

### Citizenship Status

There are approximately 22 million undocumented immigrants or individuals with legal permanent resident status living in the United States (Lee & Baker, 2017). Citizenship status can be a source of stress for clients. Given the current political climate, a client's citizenship status should be explored regarding its impact on the client's functioning. Undocumented immigrants experience a host of challenges, including fears around deportation or "being found out" that can exacerbate mental health problems (Leyro, 2015). Clients who are citizens, but from mixed-status families, may experience additional stressors and hesitation to engage in treatment (Mazzula & Torres, 2017). Therefore, the impact of citizenship status on clients must be addressed and integrated in treatment.

## Language

Language barriers are related to underutilization of metal health services, lack of patient satisfaction, poor-quality patient education, and premature termination. Language barriers can hinder effective communication between the client and the counselor. Mental health providers have been shown to have a lack of respect or interest in clients when a language barrier is present, and as a result engage in misdiagnosis and perceive clients to lack awareness of their medical problems (Arredondo et al., 2014; Mio et al., 2016; Sue & Sue, 2013). Understanding the nuances of language and their impact in treatment is critical to building rapport, engaging clients, and providing relevant services.

## Gender and Gender Roles

All people are socialized in the context of gender roles (e.g., girls wear pink and boys wear blue). Gender roles are often related to the way in which mental health problems are presented. For example, research shows reduced rates of depression among males because depression may be presented in the form of anger, substance abuse, and increased risk-taking—which tend to be more stereotypical notions of male behavior (Nadal, Mazzula, & Rivera, 2017). Counselors may misunderstand gender-inconsistent behaviors, which could lead to a misunderstanding of a client's presentation and diagnosis. For example, women are more likely to be diagnosed with depression, whereas men more likely to be diagnosed with a substance abuse disorder; this is likely due to gender differences in presentation. The *DSM* may not adequately capture the role of gender and gender norms in mental health disorders.

Gender norms may be particularly salient among some racial and ethnic minority groups. Emerging scholarship shows that female gender norms characterize Latina women as being self-sacrificing for their families (e.g., *Marianismo*). Some African American women tend to be characterized as self-reliant and solely responsible for the care of the family without support from others (e.g., *Superwoman complex* or *Superwoman syndrome*), which is different than the gender roles assigned to some Latina and Asian American women who are characterized as being more interdependent. Gender roles impact utilization of mental health services. For example, among African American women, there may be added pressures to be a "strong Black woman," which may impact a person's help-seeking behavior and engagement. Proper assessment and integration of these values by counselors is critical.

## TGNC AND LGBQ

Individuals who are transgender and gender nonconforming (TGNC), as well as lesbian, gay, bisexual, or queer (LGBQ), may be at a higher risk of developing mental health problems due to the discrimination and stigma surrounding gender identities and sexual orientations (Gary, 2005).

Throughout history, psychiatry, psychology, and other mental health fields have marginalized and stigmatized TGNC and LGBQ people. For example, the first three versions of the *DSM* categorized nonheterosexual sexual orientations as pathological and as "diseases." Originally included in the *DSM* was a diagnosis of "homosexuality," and subsequently as "Sexual Orientation Disorder," which encouraged physically invasive and harmful treatments. Despite the fact that sexual orientations of LGBQ people are normal and healthy, there are counselors who may attempt to "convert" clients to a heterosexual identity. To date, there is no empirical evidence to support the benefits of this approach; rather, evidence suggests that it only results in severe psychological distress (Nadal et al., 2017). "Conversion therapy" has recently been banned in some states due to the harmful nature of this "treatment."

We should note here terminologies that also further oppress, stigmatize, and marginalize TGNC and LGBQ communities. Heteronormative assumptions are pervasive in most Western institutions. Even in spoken English, we use the words *he* or *she* when describing people. This assumes that sex is a binary construct. Although it does not necessarily impact individuals who are cisgender (i.e., biological sex at birth matches the individual's gender identity), it fails to capture those who do not identify as such (e.g., gender fluid, gender identity is flexible; transgender, biological sex at birth does not match person's gender identity). Similarly, the word *homosexual*, though still widely used, is no longer used by many TGNC/LGBQ people or allies because it is an outdated term with connotations of clinical pathology, criminal behavior, and deviance. According to APA, using the term *homosexual* is also not ethical practice (APA, 1991).

## Racism and Discrimination

Racial and ethnic minority persons continue to experience racism and discrimination on individual, institutional, and system levels (Carter et al., 2013). Racism and discrimination are related to a host of problems, including negative outlook (Nadal, Mazzula, Rivera, & Fujii-Doe, 2014), poor infant development, unhealthy behaviors such as smoking (Lee, Ayers, & Kronenfeld, 2009), and traumatic stress reactions (Carter et al., 2013). Internalized racism also leads to poor self-esteem and mental health problems (Campón & Carter, 2015). Studies find similar negative consequences among LGBT people of color (Nadal, 2013).

Over the last decade, there has been a shift in understanding racism to include microaggressions (Mazzula & Nadal, 2015; Nadal, 2013; Nadal et al., 2014; Sue et al., 2007). These are "brief and commonplace daily verbal, behavioral, and environmental indignities, whether intentional or unintentional, that communicate hostile, derogatory, or negative racial slights and insults to the target person or group" (Sue et al., 2007, p. 273). Scholars argue that these subtler forms of discrimination are linked to many negative outcomes ranging from poor mental health (Nadal, Griffin, Wong, Hamit, & Rasmus, 2014) to poor treatment engagement (Mazzula & Nadal, 2015). Stressors related to racism and discrimination are exacerbated when intersectionality is considered (e.g., gender identities, citizenship status, social class, etc.). Proper assessment of the role of racism, discrimination, and microaggressions in clients' lives is critical, and it is equally important to incorporate these considerations into treatment planning and discussions with clients.

## Disability

People with disabilities have been discriminated against throughout history. Individuals with disabilities have been force sterilized, a procedure found constitutional by the U.S. Supreme Court in 1927 and one that remained legal in some states until recent times. It was also normal to segregate people with disabilities until the 1960s. For review, see Freedman, Martin, and Schoeni, 2004.

Resources and relevant therapeutic services for individuals with disability are scarce. Yet, whether or not counselors are trained to provide culturally competent treatment to individuals with disability, they are likely to encounter clients with disabilities (see Smith, Foley, & Chaney, 2008, for a review). Accordingly, counselors must prepare themselves to effectively work with and support this population. Counselors also need to engage in proper assessments so that they may refer to more competent counselors, should referral be needed.

## Social Class

It is well documented that social class impacts the well-being of people, in large part determining where they live, the access they have to services, and their overall life satisfaction. The intersectionality of race and class has also been widely noted, with people of color often overrepresented in poorer communities. Therefore, stressors related to race and social class are often exacerbated when intersectionality is considered. However, similar to people with disabilities or with TGNC and LGBQ people, there is very little training for counselors or materials to inform their competent treatment (Smith et al., 2008). It thus usually falls to counselors to prepare themselves to effectively understand the adverse impact that classism has on the mental health of people living in poverty. If counselors are not properly educated and trained to understand issues of oppression and intersectionality, they may not be able to effectively provide counseling to this population.

## Religion

Religion and spirituality are integral to many clients' well-being. However, members of some religions, such as Islam or Judaism, are currently experiencing specific discrimination, stigma, and stressors. Counselors must be aware of the political and cultural contexts relating to religion, as well as personal assumptions and biases they may have regarding religion. Given the prevalence of religion in many communities and in some cultural groups, counselors must be prepared to assess the impact of this variable on clients' functioning, help-seeking behaviors, and treatment engagement. However, similar to other cultural variables (e.g., gender identity, ethnicity, disability), limited research, resources, and training are available to counselors (Vieten et al., 2016). Thus, counselors must educate themselves to assess and integrate issues of religion or spirituality in treatment, and to make the appropriate referrals when necessary. Supervision and consultation are often necessary.

### ACTIVITY 5.1

Return to the case vignette you read in Chapter 2, Confidentiality, about John and Gloria. You may recall that Gloria was in a women's correctional facility, preparing to have an intake interview to determine her level of risk for suicide and the types of mental health services that would be needed. Consider the following: (a) Do you have a different reaction to the case than you did when you first read it? (b) Would your recommendations change, or would they stay the same? and (c) How would you engage Gloria if you were the counselor, given her sociocultural realities?

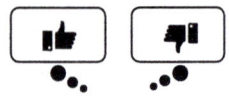

In general, counselors must ensure that all individuals receive adequate treatment that is relevant to their specific demographic characteristics and social-political realities. There are several gray areas that pose dilemmas for counselors in this regard. In this chapter, we cover two dilemmas we have encountered when attempting to engage in culturally competent treatment: (a) when worldviews collide and (b) crossing ethical boundaries. We recognize that many other ethical dilemmas related to cultural competence may also arise, some of which are discussed in other chapters of the book.

## REVIEW OF ETHICAL STANDARDS

First, let us go over where we can read about culturally competent treatment in both sets of ethical standards by the American Psychological Association (APA, 2017) and the American Counseling Association (ACA, 2014). We should note here that neither uses the term *culturally competent treatment*; rather, both use words like *cultural sensitivity*, *diversity*, and *discrimination*. Ethical codes relevant to resolving issues of cultural competence are interwoven throughout the codes of ethics. That is, neither has a specific section where you can go for answers. Therefore, it is important to untangle the ethical dilemma and know that you may need to refer to multiple codes of ethics depending on the specific ethical issue.

## APA Ethical Principles of Psychologists and Code of Conduct

APA introduces issues of cultural competence in its outline of general principles. APA's Principle D: Justice, states:

> *Psychologists recognize that fairness and justice entitle all persons to access to and benefit from the contributions of psychology and to equal quality in*

*the processes, procedures, and services being conducted by psychologists. Psychologists exercise reasonable judgment and take precautions to ensure that their potential biases, the boundaries of their competence, and the limitations of their expertise do not lead to or condone unjust practices. (APA, 2017, p. 4)*

In its next principle, Principle E: Respect for People's Rights and Dignity, APA incorporates issues of cultural competence more specifically:

*Psychologists respect the dignity and worth of all people, and the rights of individuals to privacy, confidentiality, and self-determination. Psychologists are aware that special safeguards may be necessary to protect the rights and welfare of persons or communities whose vulnerabilities impair autonomous decision making. Psychologists are aware of and respect cultural, individual and role differences, including those based on age, gender, gender identity, race, ethnicity, culture, national origin, religion, sexual orientation, disability, language, and socioeconomic status and consider these factors when working with members of such groups. Psychologists try to eliminate the effect on their work of biases based on those factors, and they do not knowingly participate in or condone activities of others based upon such prejudices. (APA, 2017, p. 4)*

Following these Principles, APA includes relevant ethical codes under various major headings. Under Competence, Code 2.01b, Boundaries of Competence, discusses the importance of ensuring that counselors have the training and experience needed to provide treatment that incorporates issues related to social-cultural identities (e.g., gender identity, ethnicity, religion, sexual orientation, disability, social class). Under the section on Human Relations, Code 3.01, Unfair Discrimination, covers refraining from discrimination toward clients based on the aforementioned social-political realities. More than one code relevant to cultural competence appears under Assessment. These codes include the use of assessment tools that are congruent with clients' backgrounds (APA 9.02b, Use of Assessments), consideration of clients' language preference and competence (APA 9.02c, Use of Assessments), and the role of culture in interpretation of results (APA 9.06, Interpreting Assessment Results).

# ACA Code of Ethics

ACA also begins its code of ethics by introducing issues of cultural diversity in the description of its professional values and principles. The second professional value is "honoring diversity and embracing a multicultural approach in support of the worth, dignity, potential, and uniqueness of people within their social and cultural contexts" (p. 3), followed by value number three, "promoting social justice" (p. 3).

According to ACA, professional values provide a conceptual basis for the ethical principles that guide ethical behavior and decision making. Two principles related to multicultural competence are Autonomy, "or fostering the right to control the direction of one's life"; and Justice, "or treating individuals equitably and fostering fairness and equality" (ACA, 2014, p. 3).

Similar to APA, the ACA code follows its description of values and principles with ethical codes under various major headings. Under Section A, The Counseling Relationship, there are two codes that are directly related to culturally competent treatment. These are Code A.2.c., Developmental and Cultural Sensitivity, which states the importance of using language that clients understand; and Code A.4.b., Personal Values, on self-awareness of personal values, beliefs, and attitudes.

Section B, Confidentiality and Privacy, begins with an aspirational introduction that states:

*Counselors recognize that trust is a cornerstone of the counseling relationship. Counselors aspire to earn the trust of clients by creating an ongoing partnership, establishing and upholding appropriate boundaries, and maintaining confidentiality. Counselors communicate the parameters of confidentiality in a culturally competent manner. (ACA, 2014, p. 7)*

Following this aspirational instruction, Code B.1.a., Multicultural/Diversity Considerations, discusses the importance of understanding cultural meanings regarding issues of confidentiality. There is also a code under Section C, Professional Responsibility, that prohibits counselors from discriminating against others based on social-cultural identities (Code C.5., Nondiscrimination; ACA, 2014) and several under Section E, Evaluation, Assessment, and Interpretation. For example, Code E.5.b., Cultural Sensitivity, focuses on cultural sensitivity when conducting assessments, and Code E.5.c., Historical and Social Prejudices in the Diagnosis of Pathology, on understanding history as it relates to the misdiagnosis of people who have primarily been marginalized populations.

As with all ethical dilemmas, there are many other codes that counselors may have to consult to inform ethical decision making, even if these codes do not directly mention issues of cultural competence. For example, ACA Code C.2.d., Monitor Effectiveness, discusses the importance of self-awareness regarding one's level of effectiveness. While broadly discussed, it has significant application to the practice of culturally competent treatment.

## DIFFERENCES AND OVERLAP

Counselors may experience a variety of ethical dilemmas related to cultural issues. Much has been written about culturally competent treatment, although not enough attention has been paid to the changing demographic characteristics of the United States. Ethical issues are complex, and even more so when we consider cultural issues.

As mentioned in Chapter 1, and throughout the book, no one sets out to be unethical. For counselors, especially, the thought that we may harm others because of our actions seems counterintuitive to our identity. However, we are all humans, socialized within our own cultural contexts. Many times we may function "normally" according to our own life experiences and training without realizing that this in itself may oppress or hurt another. In other words, it is that old saying about being a fish in water: it is difficult for fish to recognize water because they live in it, breathe it, are immersed in it, and see nothing different with which to make a comparison.

For these reasons, this chapter reviews two ethical issues which we find challenging for any counselor, given their nuances: (a) understanding how worldviews may collide and (b) what happens when boundaries are crossed. We also discuss the role of self-awareness in sound ethical decisions. We review each of these dilemmas and walk through how APA and ACA can guide our ethical decisions regarding each of these dilemmas.

### ACTIVITY 5.2

We recognize that there are many other ethical dilemmas beside those noted in this chapter. Think of ethical dilemmas you have encountered. Write them down. Return to them after reviewing the dilemmas presented here and consider the following: (a) Did I make a sound ethical decision? (b) Would I do something different if it happened again? (c) What aspects of my identity were triggered by that dilemma?

## Dilemma 1: Understanding How Worldviews May Collide

All individuals are socialized within cultural groups that have norms and values that inform the worldview of their members. These often operate on a subconscious level, and are supported by all systems in that society. Social norms and values inform the meaning that people attribute to everything—from relationships to parenting styles to help-seeking behaviors. These worldviews also inform how counselors engage clients, how they interact, and how ethical issues are navigated.

The cultural worldview of the United States is typically characterized by Western values of individuality, verbal communication, democracy, self-expression, self-actualization, and differentiation from family (Stewart & Bennett, 1991). Individualist cultural values are interwoven throughout most of our clinical theoretical orientations and approaches to treatment. For example, individual therapy is often emphasized, as is the importance of clients "speaking to us" about their feelings and issues, and of clients having the "agency" to help themselves (Mazzula & Torres, 2017). In other words, we typically value individuality and independence over collectivistic values or interdependence. This provides a very specific, and frequently narrow, understanding of human thought, behavior, affect, healing, and recovery. It is not a wrong worldview, but rather just one worldview that most counselors have been trained under.

Many cultural groups in the United States do not adhere to Western-individualistic cultural values. There are many Americans who identify with, for example, collectivist values of interdependence, cooperation, and family alliance and loyalty. From the perspective of a Western worldview, each individual person has the autonomy to engage in treatment and also to decide its course of action. Thus, this approach would typically not consider clients' family or informal support systems in treatment (Arredondo et al., 2014; Mazzula & Rangel, 2011; Sue & Sue, 2008), unless the client was in family therapy as opposed to individual treatment. Latina/o, African American, and Asian American populations are typically considered collectivist cultures.

For example, some Asian American women have been shown to see "emotional control" as a sign of strength or disclosure of problems as a way of bringing "shame" to the family. From a Western perspective, such a client could be misunderstood as having lack of insight, as hiding her emotions, or as avoiding the root of her problems. Counselors who encourage verbal expression of feelings or attempt to "dig into" the presenting problem without understanding the client's worldviews may not only be culturally inappropriate, but also pile on additional stressors for Asian American women in treatment (Nadal et al., 2017).

Similarly, many Latino subethnic groups are characterized by strong family allegiance, and help-seeking behaviors often include support from family and social support networks (Arredondo et al., 2014). We have seen this in therapy where clients spend a considerable amount of time discussing their children and family. From a Western perspective, such clients could be misunderstood as having lack of insight or unwillingness to discuss why they are in treatment. Counselors who encourage individuality, self-actualization, and differentiation from family may run the risk of adding stress and additional problems to the client. Counselors may also misdiagnose the client with attachment issues or have a difficult time "bringing in the family" when the clients are in individual therapy.

We should note here, however, that worldviews are not dichotomous. Studies show that worldviews are complex and include an intersection of other issues such as level of acculturation or racial/cultural identity (Arredondo et al., 2014; Carter, Yeh, & Mazzula, 2008).

Therefore, perhaps one of the biggest ethical dilemmas that counselors encounter is how to work with clients whose worldviews are in stark contrast to those of Western psychology. A problem arises when we use this worldview to treat others without engaging in critical thinking about its effectiveness and relevancy. However, like a fish in water, how could counselors know when their worldviews are different from those of their clients? Let us return to the ethical codes regarding competent treatment (see Chapter 4). APA's Code 2.01a-b, Boundaries of Competence, states the following:

> *(a) Psychologists provide services, teach and conduct research with populations and in areas only within the boundaries of their competence, based on their education, training, supervised experience, consultation, study, or professional experience. (b) Where scientific or professional knowledge in the discipline of psychology establishes that an understanding of factors associated with age, gender, gender identity, race, ethnicity, culture, national origin, religion, sexual orientation, disability, language, or socioeconomic status is essential for effective implementation of their services or research, psychologists have or obtain the training, experience, consultation or supervision necessary to*

*ensure the competence of their services, or they make appropriate referrals, except as provided in Standard 2.02, Providing Services in Emergencies. (APA, 2017, p. 5)*

Based on these code sections, and given professional knowledge regarding the role of culture, we could assume that "worldviews" are included in this broad mention of competence. The quoted codes mention that counselors provide services "only within the boundaries of their competence" (APA Code 2.01a) and that they "have or obtain the training, experience, consultation, or supervision necessary to ensure the competence of their services" (APA Code 2.01b). However, upon a closer look at the wording in APA Code 2.01b, you may realize that the code begins by noting that this is so when scientific or professional knowledge has established that sociocultural realties of clients are important. This creates somewhat of a problem for counselors.

First, counselors need to be abreast of current understandings of diverse populations. That means that continuing education is critical to maintaining cultural competence. However, perhaps the greatest challenge is the reality that most of the psychology research that informs theory has primarily been conducted with participants who have been Caucasian-White, male, affluent, from industrialized societies, and, many times, college students. This is a dilemma. Do all counselors even know this? Or are they the fish in water? Also, do we follow the code as explicitly written? That is, to continue business as usual when we have clients whose backgrounds have not been fully understood by mainstream psychology (e.g., Native American populations, gay, lesbian, bisexual, transgender people). Or, do we go beyond what is explicitly written in one particular code?

We should always remember the aspirations of these codes. For example, recall APA's Principle E, Respect for People's Rights, highlights that counselors know about and respect clients' sociodemographic characteristics and identities (e.g., age, gender identity, national origin, religion, socioeconomic status, etc.) and eliminate their biases. In contrast, ACA codes do not limit competence to when scientific or professional knowledge has established that sociocultural realities of clients are important. ACA's Code C.2.a., Boundaries of Competence, states:

*Counselors practice only within the boundaries of their competence, based on their education, training, supervised experience, state and national professional credentials, and appropriate professional experience. Whereas multicultural counseling competency is required across all counseling specialties, counselors gain knowledge, personal awareness, sensitivity, dispositions, and skills pertinent to being a culturally competent counselor in working with a diverse client population. (ACA, 2014, p. 8)*

ACA's Code E.5.b., Cultural Sensitivity, also notes:

*Counselors recognize that culture affects the manner in which clients' problems are defined and experienced. Clients' socioeconomic and cultural experiences are considered when diagnosing mental disorders. (ACA, 2014, p. 8)*

Now let us go a little deeper into the words *culture* as used in APA and the words *multicultural counseling* or *cultural experiences* used in ACA. Exactly what do they mean? This is often left to the interpretation and knowledge base of the counselor. Due to limited research in the areas of diversity, it is easy to miss some of the nuances. When counselors are trained from a Western perspective, which characterizes most theories of psychology, they may also come to understand how people heal, recover, and engage in treatment from this perspective—even when it is out of their conscious awareness.

Clients who have to navigate different cultural worldviews (e.g., their heritage culture and the mainstream culture of the United States), irrespective of whether they are recent immigrants or born in the United States, have to negotiate these different, and often conflicting, worldviews (e.g., interdependence vs. autonomy values). When individuals experience a pull to hold on to worldviews that are different from Western worldviews, while at the same time being pulled to endorse Western values, the conflict and tension can cause significant stress. An example is the abovementioned rise in suicide attempts among Latina adolescent girls. Research shows this is related, in part, to conflicting worldviews of the adolescent and her parents (Zayas, 2011). Similarly, when a counselor's and a client's worldviews collide, it can result in early termination and poor engagement.

According to NAMI (2009), lack of cultural competence is one of the key areas contributing to what it reported as a "dismal" state of mental health services across the United States. Counselors who understand how their clients' worldview impacts their life experiences, clinical issues, and ways of healing will help facilitate engagement in treatment, better rapport, and overall satisfaction with the counselor–client relationship.

## ACTIVITY 5.3

Although broad generalizations regarding the worldview of diverse populations are often made, there is significant variability in social-cultural identities (e.g., race, ethnicity, gender, social class, etc.) among these broad racial/ethnic categories.

This week, observe the words used by three to five individuals. They could be friends, colleagues, teachers, or family members. Take some time to write down what you hear. For example, do their conversations center around their "self"—that is, their attributes, their individual experiences, or their individual accomplishments? Or do the words used center around the "roles" and "relationships" they have—that is, their experiences as parents, students, members of marginalized groups, relationships with others? Reflect back on your answers after you have read this entire chapter.

Ask yourself if: (a) you had judgments about good vs. bad ways of conversing, (b) you can apply your learning to understand the observations you had, and (c) you changed your perception of those observations.

## VIGNETTES FOR DISCUSSION

### Instructions

Think through the ethical dilemmas represented by the following short vignettes, and answer the questions that follow as honestly as you can. Remember to monitor your reactions, keeping track of any that include shaming the counselor for "bad" behavior or for being a "bad counselor." Focus on internal and external factors that may have led to this behavior. Now is the time to notice if there are any patterns in your reactions, or the substance of your reactions, and to discuss these in supervision and consultation. This is valuable information for your reflection on what some of your personal biases and blind spots may be. (See the Appendix, Typical Cognitive and Emotional Reactions, at the end of this book.)

### Vignette 1

*A White male counselor is working in a community mental health clinic with an Asian American female client diagnosed with depression, without history of suicidal attempts. The counselor did his graduate training in the United States, but also took several courses related to multicultural psychology, so he feels competent to work with this client. The counselor also read an article that discussed Asian American populations' underutilization of mainstream mental health treatment, and therefore works really hard to engage the client to make sure that she continues with services. Over the last sessions, the counselor notices that despite his attempts to build rapport and help the client talk about her problems, she doesn't go into any depth. He also begins to feel a little frustrated because she has shown little affect and appears to be rationalizing her experience—in fact, his progress notes continue to mention how her affect is incongruent with her stated mood. The client tells him that she feels depressed, but she shows very little affect during sessions. He is concerned and consults with a colleague. His colleague tells him that the client may be out of touch with her problems or emotions and encourages him to work harder at reflecting feelings to bring those to her awareness.*

### Resolving the Ethical Dilemma

Take some time to think through the following questions. Write them down.

1. Is there an ethical dilemma here? If so, what is it?
2. Are there particular aspects of the client's worldviews that the counselor may need to explore? If so, which may those be?
3. Are there aspects of the client's sociocultural identities that the counselor may need to explore? If so, which may those be?
4. Which ethical standards would be helpful for the counselor to review?
5. Are there other ethical codes to which the counselor may need to refer to answer this dilemma?

*(continued)*

## VIGNETTES FOR DISCUSSION (continued)

6. Should the counselor seek additional consultation, training, or experience to continue working with this client? Would you consider him to be "multiculturally competent" with regard to this specific client?
7. Do you have any reactions to the vignette? If so, what are they?
8. What would you do if you were the counselor?

### Vignette 2

*A Latina counselor is working in an inpatient unit with a Latino male client who has been diagnosed with anxiety and substance use disorders. As the only counselor from a Latinx (gender-neutral term) background, and the only Spanish-speaking person, she is usually assigned all the Latinx clients. She feels comfortable with these arrangements because she can relate to the culture. As the sessions progress, the counselor begins to feel stuck. She can't get this client to talk about anything that would help her figure out what "caused" his presenting problems. Instead, most sessions focus on what his children and spouse do. While the counselor thinks it is okay for him to spend some time talking about his family, she cannot really figure out what it has to do with his problems. She also cannot get him to set goals for treatment—he simply agrees with whatever she suggests. The counselor thinks part of the problem is that he is lacking self-initiative to do things that would make him feel better and spends time talking about his family because he is in denial about his real problems, especially his substance abuse. The counselor begins to feel hopeless and thinks that she is working harder than her client and, at this point, they are just wasting time.*

### Resolving the Ethical Dilemma

Take some time to think through the following questions. Write them down.

1. Is there an ethical dilemma here? If so, what is it?
2. Are there particular aspects of the client's worldviews that the counselor may need to explore? If so, which may those be?
3. Are there aspects of the client's sociocultural identities that the counselor may need to explore? If so, which may those be? Is this counselor "multiculturally competent" to work with this client?
4. Which ethical standards would be helpful for the counselor to review?
5. Are there other ethical codes to which the counselor may need to refer to answer this dilemma?
6. Should the counselor seek additional consultation, training, or experience to continue working with this client?
7. Do you have any reactions to this vignette? If so, what are they?
8. What would you do if you were the counselor?

# Dilemma 2: Crossing Ethical Boundaries

The second dilemma is related to boundaries. As you may recall from Chapter 3, maintaining professional boundaries ensures that counselors can maintain a healthy and trusting relationship with clients. A professional boundary, in other words, is a limit on when or how we engage clients, and typically is informed by theoretical orientation, research, and standards of practice. There are boundaries that when crossed are very easy to identify as ethical violations. For example, a sexual relationship with the client is a clear violation of a professional boundary, and one that has been heavily covered in the literature.

However, there are other boundary crossings that at face value may appear to violate some ethical responsibility, but upon closer examination may not be violations given clients' worldviews and life experiences. Consider the following questions that come up for counselors related to time and invitations we may receive from our clients. Some of these questions may be explained by theoretical underpinnings, clinical, or training issues. However, focus for a moment on the role of cultural variables and social-political realities as you read the questions. When we, the authors, have similar questions, we attempt to recognize when our questions are informed by our own worldviews and values as opposed to when they are a clinical or training issue.

## Time Preference

Most counselors, irrespective of theoretical orientation, have come to know that a typical traditional individual therapy session runs 50 minutes. Given what we have been taught, both young and seasoned counselors may have reactions when this time boundary is violated.

- What do I do when my client seems to be in the moment and we are experiencing something powerful, but it is the end of the session?
- How can I just stop a client in the middle of a disclosure when we are getting to the end of the session?
- What do I do when my clients drop "cliff hangers"? That is, waiting all the way till 5 minutes before the end of the session to disclose something really important.
- What do I do if my client shows up late to my appointments?
- What do I do when my client prefers to "chitchat" about things that are irrelevant to the presenting problem (e.g., how I'm doing, how the weather is)?
- Can I tease apart motivations for the client's behavior that are clinical vs. cultural in nature, and can I tease apart my own reactions to this behavior that are based on practical attempts to maintain boundaries vs. products of my cultural norms?

## Invitations

Counselors are often socialized to think of themselves as objective beings. Part of remaining objective is to maintain clear boundaries between our professional role and what would appear to be more of the role of a friend or a family member.

- What do I do if my client brings food for me during session?
- What do I do if I am conducting in-home therapy and my client has prepared lunch or dinner for me when I arrive?
- What do I do if my client invites me to a special life event, such as a funeral, a wedding, a graduation?
- What do I do if my client wants to give me a hug when I greet him in the lobby?
- What do I do if doing in-home therapy and my client is standing in the living room ready to give me a hug as soon as I walk in?

If any of the above were to happen, what ethical codes would guide our decision to assess whether or not we were violating professional boundaries? In general, APA Code 2.01a, Boundaries of Competence, as noted elsewhere in this chapter, states that counselors provide services only within the boundaries of their competence. This, therefore, leaves the counselor in a particular dilemma as to whether a violation has actually taken place. Often this kind of question would result in the counselor seeking consultation or supervision; however, that could only happen if they have knowledge that their clients' cultural values may be informing some of these behaviors. Notwithstanding this dilemma, operating outside of one's level of competence is an ethical violation.

Western cultures tend to be future oriented, but other cultures focus more on the present, which may impact the time they arrive to sessions. Clients who are more present-oriented or focus on the relational aspects of their interactions may want to "touch base" on the counselor's life, or engage in "chitchatting" as a way to build a trusting relationship. For example, as noted earlier in this chapter, Latino clients may prefer to focus on developing relationships that are nurturing and supportive (Arredondo et al., 2014) and may not be so focused on the actual time frame we prescribe. This also brings up the issue of self-disclosure (see Chapter 3, Professional Boundaries)—that is, how much or how little counselors should share. Self-disclosure is an intentional technique with a clinical purpose (e.g., to build rapport or provide a safe environment). Having knowledge about the role of cultural worldviews in how clients interact will inform the extent to which the counselor engages in answering client questions that at times may feel like a violation of the counselor's space. When considering social-political realities, social class may also impact time of arrival if, for example, the client has to take public transportation or take kids to a family member to be taken care of while the client goes to session. Thus, counselors must account for the realities of their clients without pathologizing their behavior (e.g., labeling their behavior as "resistant to treatment"), instead understanding it in context. That, however, does not mean that counselors must change their expectations for the start and end times of a session, but rather means that they must develop a full understanding of their clients' and their own personal motivations.

In contrast to APA, ACA explicitly covers guidelines related to crossing boundaries. ACA Code A.6.b., Extending Counseling Boundaries, states:

> *Counselors consider the risks and benefits of extending current counseling relationships beyond conventional parameters. Examples include attending a client's formal ceremony (e.g., a wedding/commitment ceremony or graduation), purchasing a service or product provided by a client (excepting unrestricted bartering), and visiting a client's ill family member in the hospital. In extending these boundaries, counselors take appropriate professional precautions such as informed consent, consultation, supervision, and documentation to ensure that judgment is not impaired and no harm occurs. (ACA, 2014, p. 5)*

In general, emerging professional knowledge has come to differentiate between "boundary crossing" and "boundary violations" (refer to Chapter 3 for an in-depth review). Boundary crossings are viewed as effective methods and interventions to build rapport, engage clients, and meet clients "where they are." Boundary violations, in contrast, are instances in which crossing a boundary results in poor services or harm to the client. When considering culturally competent treatment, many counselors thoughtfully and purposefully cross boundaries, in accordance with their theoretical orientation, to engage clients and help them heal. When counselors cross boundaries, they should have sound professional knowledge and purpose regarding the action, and do so in a way that is supportive of a healthy therapeutic relationship.

## VIGNETTES FOR DISCUSSION

### Instructions

As before, think through the ethical dilemmas represented by the following short vignettes, and answer the questions as honestly as you can.

### Vignette 3

*A counselor is working in a community mental health setting. He notices that one of his clients shows up late to most appointments, and shows little remorse for taking away his precious time. He is not sure what to do, as he has clients back-to-back and cannot afford to extend the time of his sessions—although he would not mind doing so at some points. The client also begins most of his sessions with questions such as "how was your day" or "how's work going"; on some occasions the client has even commented on the counselor's appearance, noting when he looks tired*

*(continued)*

## VIGNETTES FOR DISCUSSION (continued)

*or really excited. The counselor speaks with his supervisor to explore if there are personality or clinical issues surrounding the client's lateness, and what appears to be poor interpersonal boundaries.*

### Resolving the Ethical Dilemma

Take some time to think through the following questions. Write them down.

1. Is there an ethical dilemma here? If so, what is it?
2. Which ethical standards would be helpful for the counselor to review?
3. Should the counselor seek additional consultation, training, or experience to continue working with this client?
4. Do you have any reactions to the vignette? If so, what are they?
5. What would you do if you were the counselor?
6. If we identified the counselor's and client's sociocultural identities, would your answers change? If so, how?

### Vignette 4

*A counselor is employed in a college counseling center. She is working with an undergraduate student who finds herself conflicted about how much time she is away from her family due to her schooling. Although most of her time is spent working on class projects or studying for exams, she sometimes feels "guilty" or "selfish" for focusing on herself and her goals. Though the client seems focused on her family's expectations and her role within the family, the counselor often feels the urge to encourage her to "live her own life" independent of her family's expectations. During one session, the client tells her counselor that her family is having a sweet fifteen and wants the counselor to attend. She reports that her family would "feel better" if they saw the counselor because they have expressed concerns about "what she is talking about with strangers." The client also tells the counselor that if the family meets her, they would be less worried about the client being away at college.*

### Resolving the Ethical Dilemma

Take some time to think through the following questions. Write them down.

1. Is there an ethical dilemma here? If so, what is it?
2. Which ethical standards would be helpful for the counselor to review?
3. Should the counselor seek additional consultation, training, or experience to continue working with this client?
4. Do you have any reactions to the vignette? If so, what are they?
5. What would you do if you were the counselor?
6. If we identified the counselor and client's sociocultural identities, would your answers change? If so, how?

## ACTIVITY 5.4

*Challenge yourself!* Consider the vignettes you read in this chapter. Would your reactions and interpretations change if sociodemographic characteristics (e.g., age, race, nationality, ability, etc.) or social-cultural identities (e.g., gender identity, level of acculturation) of the counselor and client were changed, or assigned when they were not identified? If so, how would they change? If not, what may explain it? How can your answers to the aforementioned questions inform your awareness of biases, assumptions, and beliefs? Remember, when engaging in critical self-reflection, there are no wrong or right answers. The important part is gaining insight into potential biases and blind spots.

# SELF-AWARENESS AND CRITICAL SELF-REFLECTION

Resolving the aforementioned ethical dilemmas requires counselors to have self-awareness of their own worldview, values, and assumptions. Remember, counselors are all socialized within historical, political, and social-cultural systems (e.g., cultural group, ethnic group, racial group, etc.). These affect how we see the world, what we consider good vs. bad behavior, and how we engage our clients. However, becoming aware of and developing a knowledge of our own values, assumptions, and beliefs is challenging.

Accordingly, it is no surprise that one of the main guidelines for cultural competence issued by the APA's "Guidelines on Multicultural Education, Training, Research, Practice and Organizational Change for Psychologists" focuses on recognizing our cultural selves in context. The guideline encourages counselors to "recognize that, as cultural beings, they may hold attitudes and beliefs that can detrimentally influence their perceptions of and interactions with individuals who are ethnically and racially different from themselves" (APA, 2002, p. 17).

The APA Code of Ethics does not directly mention issues related to self-awareness, so one must refer back to the codes on boundaries of competence that speak to adequate knowledge of those being serviced by the counselor. ACA, however, has direct guidelines. For example, ACA Code, A.4.b., Personal Values, states:

> *Counselors are aware of—and avoid imposing—their own values, attitudes, beliefs, and behaviors. Counselors respect the diversity of clients, trainees, and research participants and seek training in areas in which they are at risk of imposing their values onto clients, especially when the counselor's values are inconsistent with the client's goals or are discriminatory in nature. (ACA, 2014, p. 5)*

Similarly, ACA Code E.5.c., Historical and Social Prejudices in the Diagnosis of Pathology, states:

> *Counselors recognize historical and social prejudices in the misdiagnosis and pathologizing of certain individuals and groups and strive to become aware of and address such biases in themselves or others. (ACA, 2014, pp. 11)*

Both ACA and APA encourage counselors to continue to monitor their effectiveness. ACA, Code C.2.d., Monitor Effectiveness, states:

*Counselors continually monitor their effectiveness as professionals and take steps to improve when necessary. Counselors take reasonable steps to seek peer supervision to evaluate their efficacy as counselors. (ACA, 2014, p. 8)*

APA Principle E, Respect for People's Rights and Dignity, also mentions, albeit less directly, the importance of self-monitoring: Counselors are "aware of and respect cultural, individual and role differences" and work to eliminate biases (APA, 2017, p. 4).

Engaging in critical self-reflection on our biases, values, and assumptions can lead to a host of emotional reactions, from anger to powerlessness to denial, among all counselors, particularly when it challenges issues of power and privilege (Mazzula & Rangel, 2011; Smith & Redington, 2010). However, engaging in deliberate and critical self-reflection is perhaps the best method to ensure that counselors do not oppress, marginalize, misdiagnose, or pathologize marginalized groups. We believe that no counselor wants to intentionally harm or dismiss a client's experiences. Our responsibility is to remain open to the possibility that our way of looking at the world is just that—one way out of many possibilities—and that there are diverse ways of experiencing distress, of healing, and of moving toward recovery.

# CHAPTER DISCUSSION QUESTIONS

1. What are some steps that I could follow in order to determine whether or not I am being culturally competent?
2. What may be some blind spots that I have regarding my identities which have socially constructed power (e.g., White, heterosexual, male)?
3. What aspects of my worldview may impact how I engage clients? For example, values of individualism vs. collectivism, preference for future vs. present time orientation, values of independence vs. interdependence.
4. How can I best integrate my ethical guidelines when working in professional settings that follow a separate set of ethical standards (i.e., ACA vs. APA)?

# CONCLUSION

Counselors cannot make sound ethical decisions devoid of individual and sociocultural contexts. In this chapter we reviewed that being culturally competent includes having self-awareness of our biases and assumptions, having knowledge of those with whom we work, and being able to adapt our skills so they are congruent with the needs of the people we serve. As we saw in this chapter, a host of ethical issues can arise when we do not have the necessary training, experience, or knowledge to work with diverse populations. Here, it is most important to be aware of our various areas of privilege and biases that may negatively impact our ability to effectively interpret and respond to ethical dilemmas.

## PERSONAL INVENTORY: QUESTIONS FOR FURTHER EXPLORATION

## PROFESSIONAL EXPERIENCES

1. Can you think of a time when you struggled with how to engage clients who were different from you (e.g., in terms of race, culture, nationality, social class, religion, gender identity, etc.)? What did you do and what aspects of this experience caused anxiety or discomfort?
2. Have you identified personal red flags that would help you notice when you encounter a client's worldview that is different from yours? What are those red flags? If you have yet to identify them, what can you do to notice them in future interactions with clients?
3. Have you received specific education, training, or supervision with regard to issues of privilege, oppression, intersectionality, and sociopolitical realities?

## PERSONAL EXPERIENCES

1. Has there been a situation when you were trying to tell something important to someone and they did not see the big deal? How did that feel? What did you think about that person after that moment?
2. Has a family member or friend ever told you or asked you to do something that went against your perceptions of what is right or wrong? How did you go about resolving this?

## REFERENCES

Alegria, M., Mulvaney-Day, N., Torres, M., Polo, A., Cao, Z., & Canino, G. (2007). Prevalence of psychiatric disorders across Latino subgroups in the United States. *American Journal of Public Health, 97,* 68–75.

American Counseling Association. (2014). *2014 ACA code of ethics.* Retrieved from https://www.counseling.org/resources/aca-code-of-ethics.pdf

American Psychiatric Association. (2014). *Diagnostic and statistical manual of mental disorders* (5th ed.). Arlington, VA: American Psychiatric Publishing.

American Psychological Association. (1991). Avoiding heterosexual bias in language. *American Psychologist, 46*(9), 973–974. Retrieved from http://www.apa.org/pi/lgbt/resources/language.aspx

American Psychological Association. (2002). Guidelines on multicultural education, training, research, practice and organizational change for psychologists. *American Psychologist, 58,* 377–402.

American Psychological Association. (2017). *Ethical principles of psychologists and code of conduct* (2002, amended June 1, 2010 and January 1, 2017). Retrieved from http://www.apa.org/ethics/code/index.aspx

Arredondo, P., Gallardo-Cooper, M., Delgado-Romero, E. A., & Zapata, A. L. (2014). *Culturally responsive counseling with Latinas/os*. Alexandria, VA: American Counseling Association.

Arredondo, P., Toporek, R., Brown, S., Jones, J., Locke, D., Sanchez, J., & Standler, H. A. (1996). Operationalization of multicultural counseling competencies. *Journal of Multicultural Counseling & Development, 24*, 42–78.

Campón, R. R., & Carter, R. T. (2015). The appropriated racial oppression scale: Development and preliminary validation. *Cultural Diversity and Ethnic Minority Psychology, 21*(4), 497–506. doi:10.1037/cdp0000037

Carter, R. T., Mazzula, S., Victoria, R., Vazquez, R., Hall, S., Smith, S., . . . Williams, B. (2013). Initial development of the race-based traumatic stress symptom scale: Assessing the emotional impact of racism. *Psychological Trauma: Theory, Research, Practice, and Policy, 5*(1), 1–9. doi:10.1037/a0025911

Carter, R. T., Yeh, C., & Mazzula, S. L. (2008). Cultural values orientation and racial identity attitudes: A study of Latino college students' attitudes. *Hispanic Journal of Behavioral Sciences, 30*(1), 5–23. doi:10.1177/0739986307310505

Freedman, V. A., Martin, L. G., & Schoeni, R. F. (2004). Disability in America. *Population Bulletin, 59*, 3–33. Retrieved from http://www.prb.org/Source/59.3DisabilityInAmerica.pdf

Gary, F. A. (2005). Stigma: Barrier to mental health care among ethnic minorities. *Issues in Mental Health Nursing, 26*, 979–999. doi:10.1080/01612840500280638

Lee, C., Ayers, S. L., & Kronenfeld, J. J. (2009). The association between perceived provider discrimination, health care utilization, and health status in racial and ethnic minorities. *Ethnicity & Disease, 19*(3), 330–337.

Lee, J., & Baker, B. (2017). *Estimates of the lawful permanent resident population in the United States: January 2014*. Office of Immigration Statistics, Policy Directorate, U.S. Department of Homeland Security. Retrieved from https://www.dhs.gov/sites/default/files/publications/LPR%20Population%20Estimates%20January%202014.pdf

Leyro, S. (2015). *Legal violence: Crimmigration and the violent effects of deportation*. Paper session at the 32nd annual Winter Roundtable, Teachers College, New York, NY.

Mazzula, S. L. (2015, November). *Evaluating Latino race and culture in psychology publications: Next steps in culturally relevant scholarship*. Paper presented at the American Evaluation Association Conference, Chicago, IL.

Mazzula, S. L., & Nadal, K. L. (2015). Racial microaggressions, whiteness, and feminist therapy. *Women & Therapy, 38*(3–4), 308–326. doi:10.1080/02703149.2015.1059214

Mazzula, S. L., & Rangel, R. (2011). Cultural consideration for mental health treatment with women of color. In P. Lundberg-Love, K. Nadal, & M. Paludi (Eds.), *Women and mental disorders: Treatments and research* (Vol. 4, pp. 75–91). Santa Barbara, CA: Praeger.

Mazzula, S. L., & Torres, A. (2017). Latino trends and health policy: From walking on eggshells to commitment. In L. Benuto & W. O' Donohue (Eds.), *Enhancing behavioral health in Hispanic populations: Eliminating disparities through integrated behavioral and primary care.* New York, NY: Springer Publishing.

Mio, J. S., Barker, L. A., & Tumambing, J. S. (2016). *Multicultural psychology: Understanding our diverse communities* (4th ed.). New York, NY: Oxford University Press.

Nadal, K. L. (2013). *That's so gay! Microaggressions and the lesbian, gay, bisexual, and transgender community.* Washington, DC: American Psychological Association.

Nadal, K. L., Griffin, K. E., Wong, Y., Hamit, S., & Rasmus, M. (2014). The impact of racial microaggressions on mental health: Counseling implications for clients of color. *Journal of Counseling & Development, 92*(1), 57–66. doi:10.1002/j.1556-6676.2014.00130.x

Nadal, L., Mazzula, S. L., & Rivera, D. (Eds.). (forthcoming 2017). *SAGE encyclopedia on psychology and gender* (Vols. 1–4). Thousand Oaks, CA: Sage.

Nadal, K., Mazzula, S. L., Rivera, D. R., & Fujii-Doe, W. (2014). Racial microaggressions and Latina/o Americans: An analysis of nativity, gender, and ethnicity. *Journal of Latina/o Psychology, 2*(2), 67–78. doi:10.1037/lat0000013

National Alliance on Mental Illness. (2009). *Grading the states.* Arlington, VA: Author.

Smith, L., Foley, P., & Chaney, M. (2008). Addressing classism, ableism, and heterosexism in counselor education. *Journal of Counseling & Development, 86*, 303–310.

Smith, L., & Redington, R. M. (2010). Lessons from the experiences of White antiracist activists. *Professional Psychology: Research and Practice, 41*(6), 541–549. doi:10.1037/a0021793

Stewart, E. C., & Bennett, M. J. (1991). *American cultural patterns—a cross cultural perspective.* Yarmouth, ME: Intercultural Press.

Sue, D. W., Arredondo, P., & McDavis, R. J. (1996). Multicultural competencies/standard: A pressing need. *Journal of Counseling & Development, 70*, 477–486.

Sue, D. W., Bernier, J. E., Durran, A., Feinberg, L., Pedersen, P., Smith, E. J., & Vasquez-Nuttall, E. (1982). Position paper: Cross-cultural counseling competencies. *The Counseling Psychologist, 10*, 45–52.

Sue, D. W., Capodilupo, C. M., Torino, G. C., Bucceri, J. M., Holder, A. M. B., Nadal, K. L., & Esquilin, M. ( 2007). Racial microaggressions in everyday life: Implications for counseling. *The American Psychologist, 62*(4), 271–286. doi:10.1037/0003-066x.62.4.271

Sue, D. W., & Sue, D. (2008). *Counseling the culturally diverse: Theory and practice* (5th ed.). New York, NY: Wiley.

Sue, D. W., & Sue, D. (2013). *Counseling the culturally diverse: Theory and practice* (6th ed.). New York, NY: Wiley.

Zayas, L. H. (2011). *Latinas attempting suicide: When cultures, families, and daughters collide.* New York, NY: Oxford University Press.

# CHAPTER 6

# MANAGING SOCIAL MEDIA

In the past, what counselors did, and how or when they did it, often stayed within the confines of their offices or workspaces. Unless a counselor's actions reached the public eye by virtue of being highlighted by professional organizations or by legal forums (e.g., a lawsuit that was reported by a newspaper), for all intents and purposes it was private—that is, something shared between the counselor and the client. Similarly, counselors' private lives remained private, or as private as they chose to keep them. With the rise of technology—in particular, the rise of social media—this is no longer the case. According to Lannin and Scott (2013), counselors are now faced with engaging in "*small world ethics*—ethical acuity that requires an application of ethical principles to the increasingly interconnected and transparent world that is burgeoning from online culture" (p. 135).

We have underscored throughout the book our belief that most counselors do not intend to engage in unethical behavior. There are, however, conditions under which counselors may be more likely to make choices that lead to unethical behavior. For example, lack of training or experience can result in poor judgment or exceeding one's boundaries of professional competence (see Chapter 4). In the case of social media, a counselor's life, behaviors, and choices enter a virtual space that is accessible to all: prospective clients, current clients, employers, mentees, anyone in the world. Everything that enters the world of social media is discoverable, and this is an area in which most of us have not been properly trained.

Social media is an amazing way to communicate with friends, colleagues, and family members across the world. Counselors have the right to participate in and benefit from this way of relating to others—it would be unrealistic to think otherwise. Notwithstanding this fact, counselors and trainees must critically and thoughtfully think about how their use of social media and technology may impact their professional work (Martin, 2010), whether they are using social media as a counseling tool or for personal reasons. Rosenblum (2006) noted that may users of social media "are communicating in their virtual underwear with few inhibitions" (p. 45). In this chapter, we focus on counselors' personal use of social media platforms and how their participation may result in ethical dilemmas.

## SOCIAL MEDIA IN A NUTSHELL

*Social media* is an umbrella term that refers to websites that allow users to exchange information from the comfort of their home. These websites serve various functions, from sharing content (e.g., Tumblr), to social networking (e.g., Facebook), to allowing users to engage in live discussions (e.g., Google Hangout, Skype). Recently, a popular image was circulated throughout social media explaining the different ways in which various platforms are used (author unknown). We find this quick approach helpful in understanding the various purposes of social media platforms.

As noted in the example in Table 6.1, each platform serves a different purpose. In some platforms, posts (i.e., comments) are short; in others, long. Twitter allows only 140 characters (excluding user names), and so anything written has to meet those character limits. Therefore, words are often abbreviated and sentences are incomplete. Facebook, in contrast, allows users to create short or very long posts—a whole life story if one chooses. Social media users can extend their presence online by using **hashtags**, thus allowing anyone who follows or searches for those terms to view the post. Hashtags are preceded with a number sign (#). For example, if we were to speak about this textbook, we might create a hashtag #EthicsIsFun.

**TABLE 6.1.** Social Media: Counseling Version

| PLATFORM | SAMPLE CONTENT |
| --- | --- |
| Twitter | My counseling session was awesome |
| Facebook | "Let me tell you all the reasons why I love being a counselor" |
| Foursquare | This is where I counsel clients |
| YouTube | Watch this video of me doing a counseling session |
| Instagram | Here is a picture of me before heading to my clinical site |
| Pinterest | Here is a board with everything related to counseling and therapy |
| LinkedIn | My skills include counseling, psychotherapy, mental health |
| Groupon | Half price on materials to decorate counseling offices |
| Tumblr | Check out my latest blog about counseling |
| Google+ | Here is a hangout for counselors |
| Snapchat | Here is a quick video or picture of me reading about psychology—it will self-destruct in a few seconds after you see it |
| Skype | Here is where we can have a virtual counseling session |

If every reader were to post on social media using this hashtag, we would all be able to see the posts, even if we were not friends or following each other on social media.

> **HASHTAGS** - words or short statements that, if included in posts, can be viewed by anyone who follows or searches for those terms.

Statistics regarding usage underscore the ubiquitous nature of social media. According to Facebook, one of the most popular social media platforms, there were 1.23 billion users on a daily average at the end of 2016 (Facebook, 2017). Seven out of 10 Americans use some type of social media platform (Pew Research Center, 2017).

## Privacy Settings

Although both professional codes provide guidance regarding media and advertising, counselors can have both professional and personal accounts on social media. Neither set of ethical standards provides guidelines on how to engage personal social media accounts. The American Psychological Association (APA) explicitly separates the guidelines from the nonprofessional role of the counselor, stating that the activities that the standards address "shall be distinguished from the purely private conduct of psychologists, which is not within the purview of the Ethics Code" (APA, 2017, p. 2).

The American Counseling Association (ACA) provides some direction. ACA's Code H.6.a., Social Media: Virtual Professional Presence, states:

> *In cases where counselors wish to maintain a professional and personal presence for social media use, separate professional and personal web pages and profiles are created to clearly distinguish between the two kinds of virtual presence. (ACA, 2014, p. 18)*

If counselors have personal accounts, privacy settings can protect the counselors. Privacy settings help set and enforce parameters on who can see information, "like" posts or pictures, or comment on content shared by the user. Although a discussion of privacy settings to protect personal information is beyond the scope of the chapter, here we review basic points to remember. Most social media platforms allow users to decide who can see their information, from posts to pictures and videos. It is here that we acknowledge that many counselors would prefer to keep their private social media lives separate from their personal social media lives.

For example, with personal accounts on Facebook, individuals can set their privacy settings to "public" or "friends only." When privacy settings are set to "public," all that is shared is accessible to any user. In contrast, "friends only" allows only the user's preapproved "friends" to see the content. Counselors must still be careful, as friends of the user may "tag" pictures, posts, comments, and so on. That means that information they shared on their own pages may show up elsewhere, linked to the counselor's page.

Therefore, though a counselor may not be "friends" with a client, the client may still find the counselor's social media accounts or other online information. Facebook includes various other privacy settings, such as the ability to create lists of individual users who can access information. Other social media platforms (e.g., Instagram, Snapchat, Twitter) have similar settings that allow users to decide whether their information is public or private.

It is the counselor's responsibility to keep abreast of the various privacy settings and features that protect his or her information and to ensure that he or she does not engage in unethical or ethically compromising behaviors (Martin, 2010; see Crtalic, Gibbs, Sprang, & Dell, 2015, for review). However, even when privacy settings are appropriate and enabled, information may be accessed in other ways. Hackers can steal information. Some employers or agencies also control user information. On a more practical basis, laptops and smartphones can be lost or misplaced. Therefore, these devices and social media accounts should always be password-protected. Despite these precautions, there is always a possibility that passwords and personal information may be recovered by technology-savvy individuals. Consequently, counselors must always be cognizant of the possibility of breaches and deliberate in their use of social media.

### ACTIVITY 6.1

Speak with your colleagues, instructors, academic advisors, or supervisors about their thoughts on social media in general, and on the use of social media by counselors specifically. What do they report are the pros and cons of social media? Do their thoughts align with yours?

## BENEFITS

Social media has become a major part of people's day-to-day activity. There are various benefits to social media, including providing psycho-education to the general public, highlighting research, or promoting evidence-based interventions. The use of social media and technology allows counselors to improve their client's lives, and to reach people who would otherwise not have access to psychological knowledge. It can be a way of communicating via video counseling or text messaging. Counselors may post psycho-educational information via Twitter or Facebook. Virtual meetings or counseling sessions can take place via Google Hangout with colleagues or clients across the country—in fact, around the world.

### A Counseling Tool

As a counseling-specific tool, there are many benefits to social media. In a review of ethical issues related to social media, scholars note that communications that take place virtually may reduce anxiety and create safe spaces for clients who have been marginalized (Kaplan, Wade, Conteh, & Martz, 2011). It is also well documented that individuals with severe mental illness or those who have been discriminated against due to their sociodemographic characteristics (see Chapter 5) often experience stigma around seeking mainstream mental health services. Therefore, social media could be a powerful tool to service those who would otherwise not seek treatment. For example, in a review of ethical issues related to social media in social work, Reamer (2013) noted that social media can "humanize" the therapeutic relationship for individuals with physical disabilities. In a review of ethical issues for rehabilitation counselors, Crtalic et al. (2015) also noted that it could be helpful in engaging underserved communities that lack resources to attend counseling sessions (e.g., transportation). However, access to technology could also be a barrier for financially disadvantaged communities, further marginalizing them should counselors use social media as a primary counseling tool.

## A General Knowledge Tool

Many professional organizations, institutes, and programs have established a strong presence in social media. For example, both APA and ACA promote sharing psychological knowledge by including icons (such as Twitter, Facebook, blogs, and Google+) through which users can share information from their websites. Social media platforms are also used to promote and make information accessible during professional science meetings. Example include the APA Convention or Teachers College Winter Roundtable on Cultural Education and Psychology, with targeted user names on social media platforms such as @APAConvention and @TC_Roundtable on Twitter and other platforms.

We have also seen a rise in the use of social media to increase workforce diversity and provide relatable faces for the next generation of scholars, as in the case of the Latina Researchers Network (e.g., www.facebook.com/LatinaResearchers). Funders and institutes alike are also leveraging social media to disseminate information about funding opportunities, scholarships, and internships (e.g., National Institutes of Health Loan Repayment Program, www.Twitter.com/NIH_LRP). In essence, social media is an exciting and innovative way to communicate within this field.

# DISADVANTAGES

While we believe that social media offers exciting and innovative communication options, there are various disadvantages of which counselors must be aware.

## Generational Gaps

The first limitation of social media is related to generational gaps. In a study of 695 APA doctoral-level students and licensed psychologists, Taylor, McMinn, Bufford, and Chang (2010) found that 77% of participants had social media platforms, with more users among those younger than 30 years of age. Most younger counselors were raised in an era where social media was the norm. Therefore, communicating through social media is a natural way of life. Prensky (2001) coined the term *digital natives* to refer to these individuals, and *digital immigrants* to refer to their counterparts, noting the generational gaps that seem to exist. For more seasoned counselors, supervisors, or those in senior roles, social media may be something recently learned or difficult to master.

Amid the ever-changing modalities of social media (e.g., posting live videos), older generations of counselors may feel as if they are learning a new language. We have found that learning some of these tools can be daunting. It can also be difficult to keep abreast of new social media platforms. For example, Facebook has been around long enough to gain popularity across age groups, but other platforms, such as Snapchat, that are being used with relative ease by younger generations who are digital natives can be more difficult for older generations to navigate. Thus, there may be different expectations related to the use of social media among counselors and their clients.

Similarly, there may be different expectations regarding the use of social media as a professional tool among counselors and supervisors (Crtalic et al., 2015). Generational gaps could also shift the role of supervisors; early career counselors would be more experienced when it comes to issues related to social media usage (Taylor et al., 2010). Therefore, while some are using social media to share psycho-education with the public or to communicate with others in the field, others may not be benefiting from these tools.

## Not Just for Users

Whether counselors choose to participate in social media professionally or personally, or not at all, information about them may still be available online. Everything that is posted in social media or that has ever been online is discoverable. Clients may post about their experiences in therapy, or their thoughts about you and your work with them. We did a very quick and informal search on Twitter using the phrase "my psychologist" and found comments ranging from sarcastic, denigrating interpretations of clients by their therapists to posts about a psychologist's facial expressions that were disturbing or distracting to a client. We also found posts about the benefits of counseling or the unique strengths of a particular counselor, as perceived by clients.

Relatively little is known about the extent to which clients search for information about their counselors (Kolmes & Taube, 2016). Because of the nature of social media, if stumbled upon, content of a very personal nature may be accessible to clients. In the past, most of the ethical dilemmas relating to such details focused on appropriate versus inappropriate self-disclosure on behalf of the counselor. That has changed to a more nuanced and transparent "small world ethics" as noted by Lannin and Scott (2013). In a study that examined the use of technology to search for counselor information by 332 clients, Kolmes and Taube (2016) found that participants were able to find professional, but also personal, information about their counselors, such as details about the counselor's family members. The study concluded that security and privacy of counselors' information is compromised on the Internet.

This brings up various ethical dilemmas. As clients are potentially searching for information about their counselors, social media will have to be discussed in counseling education and training regardless of whether the counselor is an active user or not (Crtalic et al., 2015). For those who are active users, keeping up to date with privacy settings and features and securing their content is critical (Crtalic et al., 2015; Martin, 2010).

Given the lack of research and concrete guidelines on navigating ethical dilemmas related to social media, there remains some ambiguity. In the study by Taylor et al. (2010), mentioned earlier, the researchers found that participants (doctoral-level students and licensed psychologists) were cognizant of ethical issues around social media. However, many were unsure how to engage in sound ethical decision making around these issues.

# Mistakes From Youth

All counselors were once young and many may have made choices that as adults they regret, hoping, internally, that no one will ever know about them: the argument with a friend in college, the night out with friends that involved one too many drinks, or the love letter to an ex-partner that should never have been sent. It is from these real-life experiences, including mistakes, that we learn, and they make us who we are. When social media was not around, most people could hope to leave those situations behind, chalking them up as a learning experience or compartmentalizing them, never to be considered again. Unless a counselor lived in a small rural community, it would be unlikely that a client would ever know a counselor's history.

In today's world of social media, when everyone has a smartphone and may post pictures or comments about you without your awareness, this becomes problematic. Counselors in their pre-professional lives may have posted pictures or videos of potentially compromising behaviors that could impact their clients' views of them. Again, when conducting an informal search on Twitter, we found various posts by individuals we presumed were in training or hoped to enter the field of counseling one day. Tweets included posts questioning an individual's future abilities (e.g., "how will a person be a psychologist when they are bad at dealing with peoples' problems or can't express their own emotions") as well as those of a potentially more compromising nature (e.g., directly asking viewers what would happen if an aspiring psychologist's nude pictures were found in a Google search). Many posts included graphic vocabulary or content.

Again, we venture to say that there are conditions in which individuals can post content on social media that is compromising, not only personally, but also for their future as counselors. Even in the case when we have set privacy settings to allow access only to "friends," the information is still out in virtual space—to be liked by others, shared by others, and interacted with by others. Years later a client might search your name and find that love note, or that picture showing the now-counselor in a compromising way. As anxiety-provoking as this may be, it is a reality and so should be confronted as such. Counselors now, more than previously, are responsible for being mindful of their professional lives even during their private time.

As noted in Chapter 2, thinking through the following questions would be helpful when discussing client-related issues involving social media or online content. These questions are important to consider before sharing information on social media, and should assist you in examining how you would proceed should compromising online content become visible to or be discovered by your clients.

- Would you want your clients to see it?
- What would it mean for them if they did?
- What would happen if friends of your clients saw it?
- How would it impact your therapeutic relationship?
- How would you discuss this in session?
- Would you need to seek supervision or consultation to competently address this with your clients?
- Think further. What if a judge read it during a civil hearing or during a trial in which you were testifying as an expert?

One must never assume that content is gone forever—even when using social media platforms such as Snapchat, where posts, pictures, or videos self-destruct within seconds of a viewer seeing them. Everything that is on the Internet is recoverable. Therefore, every future counselor, trainee, and those active in the field must maintain a level of professionalism at all times. There's really no exception.

### ACTIVITY 6.2

Many people use Google to find out information about others. Clients may use Google to find out about you in order to decide whether they want to work with you. They may even use it to find out what you are up to after starting counseling. Employers will also look up individuals to determine if they would hire them. Take a moment to Google your name. What comes up? Does it align with how you want others to see you?

---

While both APA and ACA, in their ethics codes, provide guidance regarding social media, it is a developing area. Counselors must keep abreast of state laws and regulations that guide professional conduct (Kaplan et al., 2011; Martin, 2010) and how these impact their use of social media. They must also check state licensing boards, many of which are still developing rules and guidelines for social media communications (Kaplan et al., 2011). Professional literature regarding social media does not exist to the extent that it does in other areas. Irrespective of these limitations, ethical standards and guidelines direct our professional conduct

> **ACTIVITY 6.3**
>
> Explore the laws in your state. Investigate whether these are in line with the ethical standards you learned in this chapter, or if they are in conflict with one another (see Chapter 1 on gathering information in your state).

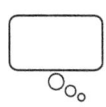

in all areas of our lives when it comes to how our actions may impact our clients. Therefore, specific training on navigating ethical issues related to social media is necessary.

As noted through the background information on the benefits and disadvantages of social media, there are various ethical dilemmas. In this chapter, we review three ethical issues and how both APA and ACA would guide our decision making: (a) whether to like, friend, or follow our clients on social media; (b) how to accurately represent ourselves on the Internet and social media platforms given boundaries of professional competence; and (c) issues related to confidentiality, as in the case of posting about clients on social media.

# SELF-ASSESSMENT: CURRENT BELIEFS AND EXPECTATIONS

## Instructions

If you were to take an essay test right now, how well would you be able to answer the following questions critically and thoroughly? Give yourself a letter grade from A to F. Be honest. There are no right or wrong questions when learning where you stand.

## Beliefs

- Role of the Counselor
    - What do you think is the role of a counselor in knowing, understanding, or incorporating social media into his or her professional life?
- Role of the Client
    - What do you think is the role of a client when it comes to issues related to social media? For example, should clients feel free to search for personal information about their counselors?
- Function of Social Media
    - What may be a benefit of using social media in counseling?
    - What may be a challenge of using social media in counseling?

## Expectations

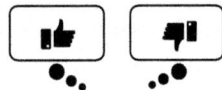

- Successes in Treatment
  - What do you think is the role of social media in communicating information regarding mental health to the public?
  - Is there a role for social media within the context of a therapeutic relationship?
- Situations That May Be Challenging
  - Identify two situations that may be personally challenging for you with regard to social media.
- Situations That May Create Ethical Dilemmas
  - What are two situations regarding social media that could realistically create an ethical dilemma for you?
- Methods for Maintaining Confidentiality
  - What could you personally do to ensure that clients are aware of issues of confidentiality as they relate to use of social media?
- Impact on Self and Professional Growth
  - What is the role of social media in your personal development as an individual and in your professional growth as a counselor who is ever-evolving?

# ETHICAL STANDARDS SURROUNDING SOCIAL MEDIA

In general, both sets of ethical standards are written very broadly, so as to be applicable to a host of diverse scenarios. The standards are not exhaustive of all ethical dilemmas. That means that neither covers every single ethical issue that may conceivably arise. This is particularly important as it relates to social media, as this area is under development. First, let us review sections where a counselor would go to read about social media guidelines in both the APA and ACA codes of ethics.

In general, most of the codes relevant to social media are grouped together. As we have emphasized throughout the book, it is always important to untangle the ethical dilemma and recognize that you may need to refer to multiple codes of ethics to resolve a single dilemma. It is no different for social media; in fact, this approach is particularly relevant, as issues related to social media may be directly linked to other codes (e.g., professional competence, as discussed later in this section).

Furthermore, it is important to note the terminology used by both APA and ACA. Whereas the ACA Code of Ethics directly mentions the term *social media*, APA tends to use words such as *Internet* and *electronic transmission*. Neither identifies social media platforms specifically (e.g., Google+, Facebook, Snapchat, Instagram, or the like). However, the spirit of these codes includes the use of social media, whether it is directly mentioned or not.

### ACTIVITY 6.4

In Chapter 1, we reviewed the importance of self-awareness in arriving at sound ethical decisions. Return to Activity 1.4 and try to answer those questions as they relate to social media. For example, one question asked if you are able to remain self-aware, or if personal or work conditions cause you to feel "shut down." Many conditions may cause counselors to feel they have shut down, including stress, overwork, and becoming jaded. Even positive emotions such as joy can cause counselors temporarily to lose sight of professional ethics and post something about their experience that may be unethical or compromising. Think through the questions honestly. This is valuable information when reflecting on your personal biases and blind spots.

## APA Ethical Principles of Psychologists and Code of Conduct

The introduction of the APA's Ethical Principles of Psychologists and Code of Conduct begins by describing the purpose and spirit of the standards. In the introduction, APA states,

> *This Ethics Code applies only to psychologists' activities that are part of their scientific, educational, or professional roles as psychologists. Areas covered include but are not limited to the clinical, counseling, and school practice of psychology; research; teaching; supervision of trainees; public service; policy development; social intervention; development of assessment instruments; conducting assessments; educational counseling; organizational consulting; forensic activities; program design and evaluation; and administration. This Ethics Code applies to these activities across a variety of contexts, such as in person, postal, telephone, Internet, and other electronic transmissions. These activities shall be distinguished from the purely private conduct of psychologists, which is not within the purview of the Ethics Code. (APA, 2017, p. 2)*

Therefore, all APA ethical codes apply to the use of social media. APA further states,

> *Membership in the APA commits members and student affiliates to comply with the standards of the APA Ethics Code and to the rules and procedures used to enforce them. Lack of awareness or misunderstanding of an Ethical Standard is not itself a defense to a charge of unethical conduct. (APA, 2017, p. 2)*

As you may notice, the APA Code of Ethics applies to all activities, including those that take place via the Internet. The last statement is particularly important given the developing nature of guidelines and standards around social media. Lack of awareness regarding the application of ethical codes to social media does not excuse a counselor who engages in unethical or compromising behaviors.

Following this introduction, APA includes ethical codes that are directly related to social media, mostly under the section related to "Advertising and Other Public Statements." These include codes related to statements made in public, whether in brochures or resumes (APA

Code 5.01a–c). An additional code can be found in this section related to conducting media presentations, such as when giving advice (APA 5.04, Media Presentations).

It is important to note here one other code that contains a direct mention: APA's Code 4.02c, Discussing the Limits of Confidentiality, which states "Psychologists who offer services, products, or information via electronic transmission inform clients/patients of the risks to privacy and limits of confidentiality" (APA, 2017).

Similarly, though not all codes directly mention social media, many codes are applicable. For example, in an interview with APA's ethics office in 2010 (Martin, 2010), it was noted that sections most relevant to social media include confidentiality and multiple relationships—these are in addition to the codes we review next that directly mention electronic transmissions. According to the interview, the code of ethics does not "prohibit all social relationships, but it does call on psychologists to ask, 'How does this particular relationship fit with the treatment relationship?'" (Martin, 2010, p. 32).

# ACA Code of Ethics

Unlike APA's Ethical Principles of Psychologists and Code of Conduct, the ACA Code of Ethics dedicates a complete section to social and electronic media: Section H: Distance Counseling, Technology, and Social Media. As you may recall from Chapter 1, ACA organizes its code of ethics by section, each beginning with an introduction that is inspirational in nature and is used to guide counselors toward the highest ideals in the practice of counseling. ACA's Section H states:

> *Counselors understand that the profession of counseling may no longer be limited to in-person, face-to-face interactions. Counselors actively attempt to understand the evolving nature of the profession with regard to distance counseling, technology, and social media and how such resources may be used to better serve their clients. Counselors strive to become knowledgeable about these resources. Counselors understand the additional concerns related to the use of distance counseling, technology, and social media and make every attempt to protect confidentiality and meet any legal and ethical requirements. (ACA, 2014, p. 17)*

Thus, ACA's Ethics Code allows counselors to use and engage in social media if this will benefit the client. However, it is their professional duty to ensure that their clients are protected and to use such media in a way that is based on sound ethical decision making.

Following this aspirational introduction, ACA includes various codes. However, unlike APA codes, which focus on public information shared by counselors in general, ACA codes focus more on guidelines that protect clients. For example, codes that directly mention the use of social media (also technology in general and distance counseling) discuss counseling-related competencies when counselors use social media for counseling purposes (ACA, 2014; Code H.1.a., Knowledge and Competency); issues, risks, and benefits that must be discussed when engaging clients in social media, in addition to general informed consent (ACA, 2014; Code H.2.a., Informed Consent and Disclosure); and informing clients about the limitations inherent in the use of social media (ACA, 2014; Code H.4.a., Distance Counseling Relationship: Benefits and Limitations).

## DIFFERENCES AND OVERLAP

Obviously, covering every single ethical dilemma that could arise with regard to electronic or social media use is beyond the scope of this book; however, we present three ethical issues that we find are potential pitfalls for counselors given the rise of technology. As previously noted, these are (a) liking, following, or friending clients on social media; (b) accurate Internet and social media representation; and (c) confidentiality. We review each of these dilemmas and walk through how the APA and ACA codes can guide our ethical decisions.

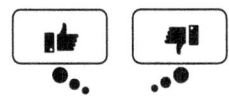

As we have noted throughout the book, we recognize that there are always additional gray areas and dilemmas that arise in the process. For example, we noted earlier APA's and ACA's stand on personal versus professional social media presence—which also may lead to various ethical dilemmas for counselors who have blurred those two.

### Dilemma 1: Likes, Follows, Friends

The first ethical dilemma surrounds the issue of whether counselors should like, follow, or friend their clients on social media, or allow their clients to do so. In short, does engaging in a virtual relationship create ethical conflicts?

APA does not provide direct guidelines on how counselors may use personal social media accounts. However, as previously noted, the introduction to APA's Code of Ethics applies to all activities, including those that take place via the Internet. Therefore, counselors must be aware of how engaging in a virtual relationship could put them at risk. One code we may review is APA's Code 3.05, Multiple Relationships, which states:

> (a) A multiple relationship occurs when a psychologist is in a professional role with a person and (1) at the same time is in another role with the same person, (2) at the same time is in a relationship with a person closely associated with or related to the person with whom the psychologist has the professional relationship, or (3) promises to enter into another relationship in the future with the person or a person closely associated with or related to the person.
>
> A psychologist refrains from entering into a multiple relationship if the multiple relationship could reasonably be expected to impair the psychologist's objectivity, competence, or effectiveness in performing his or her functions as a psychologist, or otherwise risks exploitation or harm to the person with whom the professional relationship exists. Multiple relationships that would not reasonably be expected to cause impairment or risk exploitation or harm are not unethical. . . . (APA, 2017, p. 6)

Thus, it could be interpreted that if a counselor is seeing a client and at the same time engaging in a nonprofessional virtual relationship, it would be a violation of ethical codes. When engaging in a virtual relationship for counseling-related purposes, counselors must document the rationale and receive permission from clients to do so (APA Code 3.10, Informed Consent). Therefore, as a general rule, counselors should not like, friend, follow, or allow clients to do so, unless doing so was thoughtfully considered, including benefits and risks, and for counseling purposes. Because personal accounts can include a variety of personal content, it can be assumed that being "friends" on social media would not be beneficial to the client, and also would be a violation of ethical standards.

ACA, in contrast, has several codes directly related to social media that are applicable. For example, counselors are required to create a separate and distinct virtual presence (e.g., professional versus personal, according to ACA, 2014, Code H.6., Social Media: Virtual Professional Presence). Similarly, as previously noted, counselors are allowed to use social media if it is beneficial to the client (see ACA Section H).

However, according to ACA's Code A.5.e., Personal Virtual Relationships With Current Clients, "Counselors are prohibited from engaging in a personal virtual relationship with individuals with whom they have a current counseling relationship (e.g., through social and other media)" (ACA, 2014, p. 5). Therefore, liking, following, or friending a client for noncounseling reasons is a violation of ethical codes.

## Boundary Crossing

Crossing a professional boundary can be beneficial for counseling purposes in some cases, as noted in Chapter 3, in our discussion of boundary crossings. In these instances, ACA requires counselors to consider the risks and benefits of such interactions and to document the rationale for doing so. Specifically, ACA provides the following codes:

> *ACA Code A.6.b., Extending Counseling Boundaries: Counselors consider the risks and benefits of extending current counseling relationships beyond conventional parameters. Examples include attending a client's formal ceremony (e.g., a wedding/commitment ceremony or graduation), purchasing a service or product provided by a client (excepting unrestricted bartering), and visiting a client's ill family member in the hospital. In extending these boundaries, counselors take appropriate professional precautions such as informed consent, consultation, supervision, and documentation to ensure that judgment is not impaired and no harm occurs.*
>
> *A.6.c., Documenting Boundary Extensions: If counselors extend boundaries as described in A.6.a. and A.6.b., they must officially document, prior to the interaction (when feasible), the rationale for such an interaction, the potential benefit, and anticipated consequences for the client or former client and other individuals significantly involved with the client or former client. When unintentional harm occurs to the client or former client, or to an individual significantly involved with the client or former client, the counselor must show evidence of an attempt to remedy such harm. (ACA, 2014, p. 5)*

## VIGNETTES FOR DISCUSSION

### Instructions

Think through the ethical dilemmas represented by the following short vignettes, and answer the questions as honestly as you can. Remember to monitor your reactions, keeping track of any that include shaming the counselor for "bad" behavior or for being a "bad counselor." Focus on internal and external factors that may have led to this behavior. Now is the time to notice if there are any patterns in your reactions, or the substance of your reactions, and to discuss these in supervision and consultation. This is valuable information for your reflection on what some of your personal biases and blind spots may be (see the Appendix, Typical Cognitive and Emotional Reactions, at the end of this book).

### Vignette 1

*Carlos is a counselor in a partial-care treatment facility for adolescent boys with behavioral and emotional problems. In addition to being a counselor, he is an activist with an active social media presence. He has appeared in local newspapers and writes blogs on issues of intersectionality and mental health. He sometimes talks to his clients about his blogs as a way to engage them in treatment. One of his clients, 18-year-old Johnny, found him on Facebook and sent a friend request to Carlos's personal page. Carlos thought about the request for a while and decided to accept the request. He thought it would be beneficial for Johnny to see a relatable face that was a positive role model (that's what his colleagues always tell him). He also considered the fact that most of his posts are motivational in nature; he doesn't post pictures of family members, and doesn't talk about clients.*

### Resolving the Ethical Dilemma

Take some time to think through the following questions. Write them down.

1. What is the dilemma presented here?
2. Which codes that speak to use of technology may apply to this dilemma?
3. Are there other ethical codes that may answer or bear on this dilemma?
4. Do you have any reactions to the vignette? If so, what are they?
5. If you knew that Carlos was friends with Johnny on Facebook, would this require an ethical resolution? (See Chapter 7.)

### Vignette 2

*Stephanie is a licensed professional counselor. She has a private practice where she primarily sees clients who suffer from severe agoraphobia. Stephanie uses social media to engage her clients. One of her most active social media accounts is a private Facebook group where clients can go to talk about their issues, and what she*

*(continued)*

> **VIGNETTES FOR DISCUSSION** (*continued*)
>
> *considers to be a safe place. She discusses this group with her clients, including benefits, risks, and group rules, before she sends them an invitation to join via Facebook. She has a new client, Matt, who heard about the group from a former client and sends a request to join the group. Matt has had a particularly challenging time coming to in-person counseling sessions. Although Stephanie has not had a chance to discuss this Facebook group with Matt, she decides to accept his request for two reasons: (a) he has not been able to see her in sessions and this is a way to engage him in treatment, and (b) she knows all of her clients in the Facebook group and is certain they will share the rules of engagement as soon as he joins.*
>
> **Resolving the Ethical Dilemma**
>
> Take some time to think through the following questions. Write them down.
>
> 1. What is the dilemma presented here?
> 2. Which codes that speak to use of technology may apply to this dilemma?
> 3. Are there other ethical codes that may answer or bear on this dilemma?
> 4. Do you have any reactions to the vignette? If so, what are they?

## Dilemma 2: Accurate Internet and Social Media Representation

The second ethical dilemma surrounds accurate representation on the Internet and social media platforms. Counselors are required to work within the boundaries of their professional competence. As noted in Chapter 4, issues related to professional competence include working with a clinical population without proper experience, training, and education, as well as experiencing personal or internal problems that can affect clinical work.

Let us review here the ethical codes regarding professional competence from both the APA and ACA Code of Ethics.

*APA Code 2.01, Boundaries of Competence: (a) Psychologists provide services, teach and conduct research with populations and in areas only within the boundaries of their competence, based on their education, training, supervised experience, consultation, study or professional experience. (APA, 2017)*

*ACA C.2.a., Boundaries of Competence: Counselors practice only within the boundaries of their competence, based on their education, training, supervised experience, state and national professional credentials, and appropriate professional experience. Whereas multicultural counseling competency is required across all counseling specialties, counselors gain knowledge, personal awareness, sensitivity, dispositions, and skills pertinent to being a culturally competent counselor in working with a diverse client population. (ACA, 2014, p. 8)*

APA has several codes related to information disclosed to the public. These include:

*APA Code 5.01, Avoidance of False or Deceptive Statements: (a) Public statements include but are not limited to paid or unpaid advertising, product endorsements, grant applications, licensing applications, other credentialing applications, brochures, printed matter, directory listings, personal resumes or curricula vitae, or comments for use in media such as print or electronic transmission, statements in legal proceedings, lectures and public oral presentations, and published materials. Psychologists do not knowingly make public statements that are false, deceptive, or fraudulent concerning their research, practice, or other work activities or those of persons or organizations with which they are affiliated. (b) Psychologists do not make false, deceptive, or fraudulent statements concerning (1) their training, experience, or competence; (2) their academic degrees; (3) their credentials; (4) their institutional or association affiliations; (5) their services; (6) the scientific or clinical basis for, or results or degree of success of, their services; (7) their fees; or (8) their publications or research findings. (c) Psychologists claim degrees as credentials for their health services only if those degrees (1) were earned from a regionally accredited educational institution or (2) were the basis for psychology licensure by the state in which they practice. (APA, 2017, p. 8)*

*APA Code 5.04, Media Presentations: When psychologists provide public advice or comment via print, Internet, or other electronic transmission, they take precautions to ensure that statements (1) are based on their professional knowledge, training, or experience in accord with appropriate psychological literature and practice; (2) are otherwise consistent with this Ethics Code; and (3) do not indicate that a professional relationship has been established with the recipient. (See also Standard 2.04, Bases for Scientific and Professional Judgments.) (APA, 2017, pp. 8–9)*

APA codes speak directly to the fact that providing false, inaccurate, or misleading information is a violation of ethical standards.

As noted earlier, the ACA Code of Ethics, in contrast to the APA Code, focuses more on guidelines that protect clients. These include, for example, social media–related information that counselors need to discuss when going over informed consent (Code H.2.a., Informed Consent and Disclosure; ACA, 2014). However, ACA's introduction to Section C, Professional Responsibility, begins by noting honesty and accuracy when communicating with the public. In this case, we can certainly include any information shared on social media that is open to the public.

*Counselors aspire to open, honest, and accurate communication in dealing with the public and other professionals. Counselors facilitate access to counseling services, and they practice in a nondiscriminatory manner within the boundaries of professional and personal competence; they also have a responsibility to abide by the ACA Code of Ethics. (ACA, 2014, p. 8)*

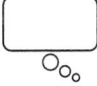

## VIGNETTES FOR DISCUSSION

### Instructions

As before, think through the ethical dilemmas represented by the following short vignettes, and answer the questions as honestly as you can.

### Vignette 3

*Clare is a doctoral candidate. Yesterday, she successfully defended her dissertation. She will be graduating once she completes this last year of internship. In her excitement about passing her dissertation, she goes to her Twitter account, @ClareJohnson (username), and tweets the following: "I'm officially a psychologist! #DissertationDone #PhD #CelebrationonTimeBeerConsumed."*

### Resolving the Ethical Dilemma

Take some time to think through the following questions. Write them down.

1. What is the dilemma presented here?
2. Which codes that speak to use of technology may apply to this dilemma?
3. Are there other ethical codes that may answer this dilemma?
4. Are there any issues here regarding professional competence?
5. Do you have any reactions to the vignette? If so, what are they?
6. If you were a counselor or colleague who saw Clare's tweet, what would you do? If anything, does it require an informal resolution or direct reporting to an ethics board? (See Chapter 7.)

### Vignette 4

*Dr. Nathan Expert received his PsyD in clinical psychology. Over the past few years, he has taken an interest in helping organizations develop their workforce by incorporating psychology to improve employee morale and productivity. In order to promote his new endeavor, he hires a social media branding company to work on flyers, brochures, and blogs he plans to disseminate in his upcoming social media campaign. To start spreading the news, he goes on his public Facebook account and posts the following to his friends: "Stay tuned for upcoming blogs on my website (www.DrNathanExpert). I strive to create positive experiences at work that promote employee happiness and satisfaction. Can't wait till you read them! #OrganizationalPsychologist #Expert #ThoughtLeader #IOPsych"*

(Note: Hashtag #IOPsych is used to refer to Industrial-Organizational Psychology.)

*(continued)*

> **VIGNETTES FOR DISCUSSION (*continued*)**
>
> ### Resolving the Ethical Dilemma
>
> Take some time to think through the following questions. Write them down.
>
> 1. What is the dilemma presented here?
> 2. Which codes may apply to this dilemma?
> 3. Are there other ethical codes to which you may need to refer to answer this dilemma?
> 4. Are there any issues here regarding professional competence?
> 5. Do you have any reactions to the vignette? If so, what are they?
> 6. If you were a counselor or colleague who saw this post, what would you do? If anything, does it require an informal resolution or direct reporting to an ethics board? (See Chapter 7.)

# Dilemma 3: Confidentiality

Confidentiality is arguably the most basic ingredient in successful therapeutic relationships. Clients must trust that their information is safe with their counselors in order to fully engage in the therapeutic process. Thus, the last ethical dilemma we discuss surrounds issues of confidentiality.

As you may recall from Chapter 2, the APA's Code 4.01, Maintaining Confidentiality, states,

> *Psychologists have a primary obligation and take reasonable precautions to protect confidential information obtained through or stored in any medium, recognizing that the extent and limits of confidentiality may be regulated by law or established by institutional rules or professional or scientific relationship. (See also Standard 2.05, Delegation of Work to Others.) (APA, 2017, p. 7)*

According to the aspiration in the introduction to ACA's Section A, The Counseling Relationship,

> *Counselors recognize that trust is a cornerstone of the counseling relationship. Counselors aspire to earn the trust of clients by creating an ongoing partnership, establishing and upholding appropriate boundaries, and maintaining confidentiality. (ACA, 2014, p. 4)*

Both sets of standards agree that counselors must protect their client's confidential information and only release it when there are good legal or ethical reasons to do so (see ACA B.1.b., Respect for Privacy; ACA B.1.c., Respect for Confidentiality; APA 4.04, Minimizing Intrusions on Privacy; APA 4.05a, Disclosures), unless prohibited by the law.

With the ubiquitous nature of social media, the potential to breach client confidentiality is grave. Anything related to your clients that is shared electronically or via social media can be considered part of the client's record (Martin, 2010). In addition, it is difficult to know who is on the other side of the computer screen. For example, consider counseling sessions over Google Hangout. Although one person is visible onscreen, it is unlikely that the counselor will be able to see who else is in the room. Consider the same scenario in the case of domestic violence. Suppose the counselor mentions something about the abuser while the counseling session is taking place—and just then that person walks in the room. There are a host of other scenarios in which breach of confidentiality is a risk. Therefore, counselors must always keep issues of confidentiality in the forefront, as well as any state laws and regulations.

Both sets of standards discuss confidentiality in the context of the Internet and social media, whether directly or indirectly. APA's Code 4.02c, Discussing the Limits of Confidentiality, states: "Psychologists who offer services, products, or information via electronic transmission inform clients/patients of the risks to privacy and limits of confidentiality" (APA, 2017, p. 7). Although APA mentions confidentiality in the context of electronic transmissions more broadly, ACA has codes that directly speak to social media and confidentiality.

> *ACA Code H.4.a., Distance Counseling Relationship: Benefits and Limitations: Counselors inform clients of the benefits and limitations of using technology applications in the provision of counseling services. Such technologies include, but are not limited to, computer hardware and/or software, telephones and applications, social media and Internet-based applications and other audio and/or video communication, or data storage devices or media.*
>
> *H.6.b., Social Media: Informed Consent: Counselors clearly explain to their clients, as part of the informed consent procedure, the benefits, limitations, and boundaries of the use of social media.*
>
> *H.6.c., Client Virtual Presence: Counselors respect the privacy of their clients' presence on social media unless given consent to view such information.*
>
> *H.6.d., Use of Public Social Media: Counselors take precautions to avoid disclosing confidential information through public social media. (ACA, 2014, p. 18)*

## To Search or Not to Search

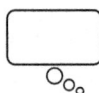

In addition to counseling-related issues, a potential disadvantage of social media is the readily available information counselors may have about their clients. In a study involving 315 counseling and psychology graduate students, Harris and Robinson Kurpis (2014) found that approximately a third used the Internet to search for information about their clients. In addition, the researchers found that the majority of those who searched for client information did so without obtaining informed consent. Counselors have the ethical duty to inform their clients about activities that directly involve them. Both ACA and APA codes (APA Code 4., Privacy and Confidentiality; ACA Code B.7.a., Respect for Privacy, respectively) state that counselors respect their clients' privacy and confidentiality. Therefore, this is an ethical violation and counselors are highly discouraged from engaging in such searches.

## VIGNETTES FOR DISCUSSION

### Instructions

Again, think through the ethical dilemmas represented by the following short vignettes, and answer the questions as honestly as you can.

### Vignette 5

*Dr. Jennifer Math is a psychologist who has worked extensively with adult clients who have a history of substance abuse problems. She has been counseling clients for more than 20 years and is known for her excellent work. After one particularly challenging session, Dr. Math goes on to her personal Facebook page, which has only a select number of friends, most of whom are family members, to take her mind off work. While looking through her friends' posts, she finds an article on substance abuse. The article addresses the challenges of working with this population. Some of the things mentioned denigrate the population, pathologize them, and emphasize negative characteristics, such as being manipulative. She decides to share the article on her page with the following statement: "There are days when I can totally relate. Today was one of them."*

### Resolving the Ethical Dilemma

Take some time to think through the following questions. Write them down.

1. What is the dilemma presented here?
2. Which codes may apply to this dilemma?
3. Are there other ethical codes to which you may need to refer to answer this dilemma?
4. Are there any issues here regarding professional competence?
5. Do you have any reactions to the vignette? If so, what are they?
6. If you were a counselor or colleague who saw this post, what would you do? If anything, does it require an informal resolution or direct reporting to an ethics board? (See Chapter 7.)

### Vignette 6

*Mary Class is a psychology doctoral student. She is teaching undergraduates in the Introduction to Psychology course as part of her teaching assistantships. During class, one of her students acts in a way that calls to mind a celebrity figure who has been in the news for various missteps. After class, she goes to her public Twitter account (@Mary Class username) and tweets the following: "One of my students is impersonating X: Please someone help, jail would not be good. #teachersproblems." (Sample post drawn from public posts.)*

### Resolving the Ethical Dilemma

Take some time to think through the following questions. Write them down.

1. What is the dilemma presented here?
2. Which codes may apply to this dilemma?

*(continued)*

## VIGNETTES FOR DISCUSSION (continued)

3. Are there other ethical codes to which you may need to refer to answer this dilemma?
4. Are there any issues here regarding professional competence?
5. Do you have any reactions to the vignette? If so, what are they?
6. If you were a counselor or colleague who saw this post, what would you do? If anything, does it require an informal resolution or direct reporting to an ethics board? (See Chapter 7.)

### Case Study 3

*Amy is a master's-level student in a licensed, eligible, professional mental health counseling program. As part of her externship, she is conducting assessments of adult clients with cognitive impairment at a local community agency. As she is drafting the results of one of her assessments to submit to her supervisor, Amy realizes she failed to find out information about neighborhood characteristics, which she thinks may have something to do with a particular client's reported history of lack of access to services. She decides to search the Internet to learn more about her client's neighborhood and, in the process, Googles the client's name. While on the Internet, she has Facebook opened and posts the following comment: "At internship site. Can't make this stuff up. Client said he can't think straight b/c his legs hurt! OMG #loveassessmentsbut #futurecounselor #counselingfunnies."(Sample post drawn from public posts.)*

### Resolving the Ethical Dilemma

Take some time to think through the following questions. Write them down.

1. What is the dilemma presented here?
2. Which codes may apply to this dilemma?
3. Are there other ethical codes to which you may need to refer to answer this dilemma?
4. Are there any issues here regarding professional competence?
5. Do you have any reactions to the vignette? If so, what are they?
6. If you were a counselor or colleague who saw this post, what would you do? If anything, does it require an informal resolution or direct reporting to an ethics board? (See Chapter 7.)

## ACTIVITY 6.5

Discussing the feelings that we are having in reaction to a colleague's, supervisor's, or instructor's use of social media can make us feel uncomfortable. Explore how you create conditions in which you would be comfortable enough to discuss your reactions. Which conditions would make this difficult? Can you create a situation with your colleagues, supervisors, instructors, or peers in which they would be comfortable sharing their personal reactions with you?

# CONCLUSION

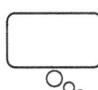

Social media has become, and likely will continue to be, an integral way in which people communicate. The potential to leverage social media for counseling-related purposes is promising. However, given the laws, rules, and ethical guidelines and standards that are still under development, counselors must proceed with caution, even when social media is used for professional purposes, and thoughtfully consider the risks and benefits. Given the interconnected, transparent, and discoverable nature of social media, personal use must also be thoughtful and deliberate.

## PERSONAL INVENTORY: QUESTIONS FOR FURTHER EXPLORATION

## PROFESSIONAL EXPERIENCES

1. Have you had an experience in the past in which a supervisor, colleague, or instructor seemed to step out of line when using social media? Can you recall what you thought or felt in response? Discussing the feelings that we are having in reaction to a colleague's, supervisor's, or instructor's use of social media can make us feel uncomfortable. Explore how you could create conditions in which you would be comfortable enough to discuss your true reactions. Which conditions would make this difficult? Can you create a situation with your peers in which they would be comfortable sharing their personal reactions with you?

2. Have you used social media for counseling-related activities? What have been the pros and cons? If you could make recommendations for others who are thinking of using social media for professional purposes, what would they be? If you haven't used social media, what do you think the pros and cons would be for you, after what you learned in this chapter?

## PERSONAL EXPERIENCES

1. If you have a personal social media account, what are your privacy settings? Do you know what resources you need to know to protect your personal information from going public?

2. If you have a personal social media account, can you think of a post you would not want a client to see? What would happen if somehow a client happened to find it? What would you say to the client who found this information?

3. Do you remember a time when a friend, who is also a counselor or counselor-in-training, posted something that gave you a knee-jerk reaction? This might have been a blog, a tweet, a video, a Facebook message, or any other form of social media communication. If so, can you recall what caused the reaction? Can you create a situation with your peers in which they would be comfortable sharing their personal reactions about your social media use?

# REFERENCES

American Counseling Association. (2014). *2014 ACA code of ethics*. Retrieved from https://www.counseling.org/resources/aca-code-of-ethics.pdf

American Psychological Association. (2017). *Ethical principles of psychologists and code of conduct* (2002, amended June 1, 2010 and January 1, 2017). Retrieved from http://www.apa.org/ethics/code/index.aspx

Crtalic, A. K., Gibbs, R. L., Sprang, M. E., & Dell, T. F. (2015). Boundaries with social media: Ethical considerations for rehabilitation professionals. *Journal of Applied Rehabilitation Counseling, 46*(3), 44–50.

Facebook. (2017). Company info: Stats. Retrieved from http://newsroom.fb.com/company-info

Harris, S., & Robinson Kurpis, S. (2014). Social networking and professional ethics: Client searches, informed consent, and disclosure. *Professional Psychology: Research and Practice, 45*(1), 11–19.

Kaplan, D. M., Wade, M. E., Conteh, J. A., & Martz, E. T. (2011). Legal and ethical issues surrounding the use of social media in counseling. *Counseling and Human Development, 43*(8), 1–11.

Kolmes, K., & Taube, D. O. (2016). Client discovery of psychotherapist personal information online. *Professional Psychology: Research and Practice, 47*(2), 147–154.

Lannin, D. G., & Scott, N. A. (2013). Social networking ethics: Developing best practices for the new small world. *Professional Psychology: Research and Practice, 44*(3), 135–141. doi:10.1037/a0031794

Martin, S. (2010). The internet's ethical challenges: Should you google your clients? Should you "friend" a student on Facebook? APA's Ethics Director Stephen Behnke answers those questions and more. *Monitor, 41*(7), 32.

Pew Research Center. (2017). Social networking fact sheet. Retrieved from http://www.pewinternet.org/fact-sheet/social-media

Prensky, M. (2001). Digital natives, digital immigrants. *Horizon, 9*(5), 1–6. doi:10.1108/10748120110424816

Reamer, F. G. (2013). Social work in a digital age: Ethical and risk management challenges. *Social Work, 58*(2), 163–172. doi: 10.1093/sw/swt003

Rosenblum, D. (2006). What anyone can know: The privacy risks of social networking sites. *IEEE Security and Privacy, 5*, 40–49. doi:10.1109/MSP.2007.75

Taylor, L., McMinn, M. R., Bufford, R. K., & Chang, K. B. T. (2010). Psychologists' attitudes and ethical concerns regarding the use of social networking web sites. *Professional Psychology: Research and Practice, 41*, 153–159. doi:10.1037/a0017996

# CHAPTER 7

# CONFRONTING COLLEAGUES AND OTHER STICKY SITUATIONS

We hold a serious responsibility for maintaining a sense of integrity for the profession. In order to uphold our responsibility to work toward excellence as individuals, and as a field, counselors must hold their colleagues to the same high and ethical standards. Social pressures which are produced by workplace and cultural norms (discussed in Chapter 3 on professional boundaries) may impact our ability and willingness to confront colleagues when we notice that they are not performing adequately. For example, the cohesiveness of the group within the workplace and the culture of protection or attitudes toward whistle-blowing are workplace norms that can affect one's openness to addressing concerning or problematic behaviors. Cultural norms that impact our understanding of power and authority may also impact our response to unethical behavior.

*Note:* Within this chapter, the term *confront* is used synonymously with *address.*

Just as we are responsible for identifying and responding to our own issues or shortcomings, we are also required to acknowledge and address issues when colleagues may be adversely affecting their clients. The American Psychological Association's Ethical Principles of Psychologists and Code of Conduct and the American Counseling Association's Code of Ethics provide standards for how to respond to unethical behavior in our colleagues.

In some instances there are opportunities for informal resolutions, whereas other actions will require direct reporting to leadership within a company or the state's ethics board. However, training often omits practical methods for how to address concerns regarding a colleague's behavior in a way that is both appropriate and respectful of the social structure. For example, a counselor may notice a supervisor engaging in unethical behavior. Similarly, a counselor may notice or become aware of unethical behavior by a colleague—at times, it may be a colleague who is also a friend outside of work. These circumstances will most likely naturally produce some anxiety and confusion regarding how to proceed. Rice (2015) stated that

> *peer-reporting, often considered a special case of whistleblowing, is the lateral reporting of a professional peer, either internally or to a superior, or externally*

*to an outside entity. Because peer-reporting challenges peer behavior, it can be affected by and impact in-group relationships and values. (p. 298)*

Rice identified individual factors such as biases and status; situational factors such as consequences of reporting and the type of ethical concern; and organizational factors such as culture, trust, and the propensity toward whistle-blowing that influence peer-reporting. Rice recommended that psychologists engage in "open discussions of ethical concerns" in order to avoid the dilemmas from escalating, as well as a "collective responsibility" that could reduce the pressure upon individual psychologists. Creating a support system that can provide regular consultation regarding ethical issues is a preventative method for avoiding ethical violations (Brennan, 2013).

How do counselors become aware of a colleague's potentially unethical behavior? Some methods for acquiring this information include third-party reports (through a client who was previously treated by this professional or another third party), by directly observing behavior, or by being told about the behavior by the colleague himself or herself. A colleague's incompetence or unethical behavior can cause problems in the work environment, along with problems for those with whom they work professionally.

Beginning in graduate school or early work experiences, we can all likely recall instances in which we noticed behavior by a colleague that was concerning to us. Graduate students may have observed a professor displaying problems with professional competence. Furr and Brown-Rice (2016) found that students were aware of their educators' problems with professional competence, including unprofessional behavior, inadequate supervision skills, inappropriate boundaries, and inability to regulate emotions. They also reported problems with cultural competence or cultural insensitivity, all of which resulted in resentment toward the educators. Olson, Brown-Rice, and Keller (2016) found that 69% of licensed mental health providers had noticed problems with professional competence in a colleague within their place of employment. The observed problems with professional competence included inadequate clinical skills, inability to regulate emotions, psychological dysfunction, personality disorder, substance use disorder, and unethical behavior. The authors reported that their participants believed this behavior was disrupting their work and negatively affecting client care.

Regarding a counselor becoming aware of a colleague's unethical behavior, Gladding (2013) stated that "by condoning or ignoring a situation they risk eroding their own sense of moral selfhood and find it easier to condone future ethical breaches, a phenomenon known as the 'slippery slope'" (p. 65). Gladding makes an important point, which is that not addressing a colleague's behavior has implications not only for society and the community in which that colleague is working, but also for ourselves. If we wish to maintain consistent ethical behavior regardless of the circumstances, then we must be attentive and responsive to violations by others.

If we ignore others' behaviors, then we are sure to ignore some of our own. Additionally, we must create an atmosphere in which we are open to feedback regarding our actions. If we are not receptive to feedback, then our colleagues will certainly struggle to remain receptive following our lack of openness. We must create a culture of connection around ethical dilemmas so that we can remain open and motivated to acknowledge and respond to any ethical concerns, whether they are our own or those of a colleague.

Herlihy and Dufrene (2011) surveyed expert opinions regarding current ethical issues. They found that the experts believed that "ensuring that counselors practice ethically and abide by the code" (p. 7) was the most important emerging ethical issue in counseling. They mentioned concerns that most ethical issues go unaddressed and unreported. Consistent with the experts' concerns, they also identified ethical decision making as "the most important issue in counselor preparation" (p. 9).

# COMMON DILEMMAS

In this chapter we review multiple vignettes that provide examples of complex ethical dilemmas involving clients and colleagues. The chapter discusses ethical standards that are directly related to addressing unethical behaviors. We focus on three specific gray areas that pose dilemmas for counselors. First, and perhaps one of the greatest dilemmas, is how to tell the difference between actions that can be addressed informally versus actions that require reporting to ethics committees. While discussing the importance of addressing colleagues' behaviors, it is essential to develop the ability to receive feedback ourselves. Therefore, two additional gray areas arise. First, how do we proceed when workplace rules seem to differ from our code of conduct? Second, how should we proceed if the counselor engaging in unethical behavior is a supervisor or someone in a leadership position? We review each of these gray areas and walk through how the American Psychological Association (APA) and the American Counseling Association (ACA) can guide sound ethical decisions. The chapter reviews ethical standards directly related to confronting colleagues and dealing with uncomfortable—"sticky"—situations. However, it will also rely on other ethical codes and standards mentioned throughout the textbook.

# SELF-ASSESSMENT: CURRENT BELIEFS AND EXPECTATIONS

## Instructions

If you were to take an essay test, how well would you be able to answer the following questions critically and thoroughly? Give yourself a letter grade from A to F. Be honest. There are no right or wrong answers questions when learning where you stand.

# Beliefs Regarding Confronting Colleagues

- Role of the Counselor
    - What do you think is the role of a counselor in addressing a colleague's behaviors? You may think about what your role does and does not consist of, as well as what you believe your responsibilities are.
    - What is the responsibility of the counselor regarding a colleague's noticeable decline in mental health or performance?
    - What is the responsibility of a counselor in maintaining effective working relationships with colleagues?
- Role of the Client
    - What is the responsibility of a client in providing information regarding the ethical behavior of a current, or former, counselor?
    - What are your expectations of how a client should respond to unethical behavior?
- Function of Holding Colleagues to a High Standard
    - What may be some benefits of acknowledging and acting on the importance of holding one another accountable?
    - About what issues do you feel competent in your ability to communicate ethical concerns to colleagues?
    - What personal factors may impede your ability to accurately identify issues with colleagues and/or respond to them?
    - What may be some cultural or situational variables that could impact your ability to effectively address a colleague's behavior?

# Expectations

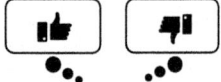

- Successes in Treatment
    - What do you think the role of confronting colleagues may be in the success of treatment?
- Situations That May Be Challenging
    - In general, which types of situations or environments would create challenges for maintaining your responsibility to report unethical behavior?
- Situations That May Create Ethical Dilemmas
    - What are two situations that would *likely* create an ethical dilemma for you when dealing with issues related to colleagues or supervisors?

- Think about your personal experience and background in noticing unethical behavior or being confronted regarding your own unethical behavior. How might these past experiences impact your reactions to current or future ethical dilemmas?
- Methods for Creating an Environment That Promotes Open Discussions of Ethical Concerns
  - What do you actively do to create an open and productive atmosphere in which you and your colleagues can freely discuss ethical concerns? Think of immediate and ongoing actions as well as your inner processes.

# ETHICAL STANDARDS SURROUNDING CONFRONTING COLLEAGUES' BEHAVIOR

First, it is important to understand where one can read about issues relating to addressing and possibly reporting ethical violations. Both APA and ACA provide standards for addressing unethical behavior in colleagues, as well as references to conflicts between organizational demands and ethical standards.

In the APA Code of Ethics (2017), Standard 1 is dedicated to "Resolving Ethical Issues." There you will find direction regarding Conflicts Between Ethics and Law, Regulations or Other Governing Legal Authority (1.02), Conflicts Between Ethics and Organizational Demands (1.03), Informal Resolution of Ethical Violations (1.04), Reporting Ethical Violations (1.05), and Cooperating with Ethics Committees (1.06).

In the ACA Code of Ethics (2014), Standard I.1: Standards and Law includes Ethical Decision Making (I.1.b.), and Conflicts Between Ethics and Laws (I.1.c.). Standard I.2: Suspected Violations includes Informal Resolution (1.2.a.), Reporting Ethical Violations (1.2.b.), Organizational Conflicts (1.2.d.), Employer Policies (D.1.g.), and Negative Conditions (D.1.h.).

Depending on the apparent ethical issue you are trying to resolve, you may find references to our responsibility to address a colleague's unethical behavior in multiple areas in the code of ethics. Therefore, it remains important to untangle the dilemma and recognize the need to refer to multiple codes, as well as the principles that are outlined in the codes of ethics.

We should also note here that as with all ethical dilemmas, other ethical issues may arise as you work through the dilemma. Not all related ethics codes will directly address the issue. Therefore, it is always important to remember that you may have to review other sections of the ethics code, not directly addressed by ACA, APA, or in this chapter, to arrive at sound ethical decisions.

### ACTIVITY 7.1

We recognize that there are many ethical dilemmas that may relate to confronting colleagues. **Think** of times when you may have felt that a colleague was doing something that didn't feel right to you. Write down what you thought was wrong with your colleague's behavior. As you read the chapter, see if you can apply some of the ethical codes and standards discussed in this chapter, or beyond, to your colleague's behavior.

## APA's Ethical Principles of Psychologists and Code of Conduct

APA (2017) provides standards for counselors who become aware of unethical behavior by colleagues. APA's Ethical Principles of Psychologists and Code of Conduct gives direction for understanding the option for an informal resolution versus the need to report the behavior to an ethics board. The APA Standard on Informal Resolution of Ethical Violations (1.04) states:

> *When psychologists believe that there may have been an ethical violation by another psychologist, they attempt to resolve the issue by bringing it to the attention of that individual, if an informal resolution appears appropriate and the intervention does not violate any confidentiality rights that may be involved. (See also Standards 1.02, Conflicts Between Ethics and Law, Regulations, or Other Governing Legal Authority, and 1.03, Conflicts Between Ethics and Organizational Demands.) (APA, 2017, p. 4)*

## ACA's Code of Ethics

ACA's Code of Ethics introduces issues of confronting colleagues under Section I, Resolving Ethical Issues, which states:

> *Professional counselors behave in an ethical and legal manner. They are aware that client welfare and trust in the profession depend on a high level of professional conduct. They hold other counselors to the same standards and are willing to take appropriate action to ensure that standards are upheld. Counselors strive to resolve ethical dilemmas with direct and open communication among all parties involved and seek consultation with colleagues and supervisors when necessary. Counselors incorporate ethical practice into their daily professional work and engage in ongoing professional development regarding current topics in ethical and legal issues in counseling. Counselors become familiar with the ACA Policy and Procedures for Processing Complaints of*

### ACTIVITY 7.2

In Chapter 1, we reviewed the importance of self-awareness in arriving at sound ethical decisions. Return to Activity 1.3 and try to answer those questions as they relate to what you learned in this chapter. For example, what aspects of your personality are triggered by the idea of "telling on" or reporting a colleague? Are you aware of your identities that have socially constructed power (e.g., White, heterosexual, affluent, native English speaker) that may impact how you resolve sticky situations?

*Ethical Violations and use it as a reference for assisting in the enforcement of the* ACA Code of Ethics. *(ACA, 2014, pp. 18–19)*

## DIFFERENCES AND OVERLAP

Both the APA and ACA codes provide standards for ways to address colleagues' apparent unethical behavior, as noted earlier, with responses ranging from an informal resolution to an official report to an ethics board. Both also acknowledge the need to protect confidentiality when considering how to respond to a colleague's unethical behavior.

## Dilemma 1: Confronting Colleagues—Choosing an Informal Versus a Formal Resolution

Choosing any form of response to a colleague's unethical or inappropriate behavior can feel challenging. Some obstacles that counselors experience for not addressing a colleague's behavior may be:

- Discomfort
- Guilt
- Anxiety
- Fear
- Confusion or lack of clarity regarding the potential violation

What does each ethics code direct us to do when we become aware of unethical or seemingly inappropriate behavior on the part of a colleague? APA has two ethical principles that seem to apply directly to these types of issues. APA's Principle of Beneficence and Nonmaleficence states:

*Psychologists strive to benefit those with whom they work and take care to do no harm. In their professional actions, psychologists seek to safeguard the welfare and rights of those with whom they interact professionally and other affected persons, and the welfare of animal subjects of research. When conflicts occur among psychologists' obligations or concerns, they attempt to resolve these conflicts in a responsible fashion that avoids or minimizes harm. Because psychologists' scientific and professional judgments and actions may affect the lives of others, they are alert to and guard against personal, financial, social, organizational, or political factors that might lead to misuse of their influence. Psychologists strive to be aware of the possible effect of their own physical and mental health on their ability to help those with whom they work. (APA, 2017, p. 3)*

This principle provides clear expectations for maintaining our own ethical behavior and for holding our colleagues responsible to do the same. It also provides the instruction to resolve ethical conflicts and concerns, taking into account internal and external variables that may impact our professional practice.

Following this principle, APA's Principle B, on Fidelity and Responsibility, states:

*Psychologists establish relationships of trust with those with whom they work. They are aware of their professional and scientific responsibilities to society and to the specific communities in which they work. Psychologists uphold professional standards of conduct, clarify their professional roles and obligations, accept appropriate responsibility for their behavior, and seek to manage conflicts of interest that could lead to exploitation or harm. Psychologists consult with, refer to, or cooperate with other professionals and institutions to the extent needed to serve the best interests of those with whom they work.* They are concerned about the ethical compliance of their colleagues' scientific and professional conduct [emphasis added]. *Psychologists strive to contribute a portion of their professional time for little or no compensation or personal advantage. (APA, 2017, p. 3)*

The quoted principle outlines the importance of establishing and maintaining trust, directly mentioning the need for attending to colleagues' professional conduct. Thus, according to APA's standard on **informal resolution** of ethical violations, when counselors become aware that another counselor is engaging in unethical behavior, they have the responsibility to bring this to the attention of that person.

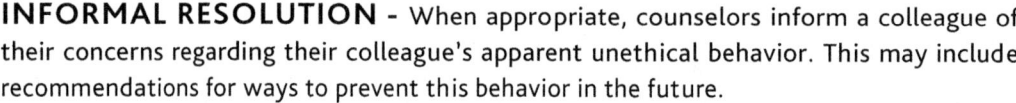

**INFORMAL RESOLUTION** - When appropriate, counselors inform a colleague of their concerns regarding their colleague's apparent unethical behavior. This may include recommendations for ways to prevent this behavior in the future.

**FORMAL RESOLUTION** - When necessary, a counselor makes a formal complaint against another mental health professional to the state ethics board or the organization in which the counselor is employed.

ACA has a similar aspiration. For example, as described under "Resolving Ethical Issues," noted earlier, counselors "hold other counselors to the same standards and are willing to take appropriate action to ensure that standards are upheld. Counselors strive to resolve ethical dilemmas with direct and open communication among all parties involved . . . ." (ACA, 2014, pp. 18–19). This can raise a host of emotional reactions for the counselor who needs to undertake the confrontation. However, it is our ethical duty to do so.

It is difficult to present concrete examples of actions that warrant an informal resolution. Many variables should be taken into consideration, such as the ethical code that was violated, who the client population is and if harm occurred, if the colleague is someone in training or someone in a leadership position who also recommends this form of inappropriate behavior, and if the colleague appears to be engaging in a pattern of behavior or this was an isolated incident. For example, a colleague may be discussing a case during group supervision and inappropriately share the client's first name. In this instance, a peer should inform the colleague of the breach of confidentiality and remind him or her that supervision should occur without any identifying information (see Chapter 2). In this instance, the risk of harm was relatively low and likely indicated the colleague's lack of clarity regarding the rule, or was an instance of a mistake. This gave the colleague an opportunity to correct the behavior so that it would not eventually reach the level of an ethical violation that should result in a formal report.

Discussing concerns with colleagues about their behavior is an inherently challenging task due to cultural norms such as "minding our own business" or not reprimanding a colleague with whom we are friendly. Judging, punishing, or attempting to police our colleagues seems to run contrary to our training as counselors (Remley & Herlihy, 2014). Therefore, we must seek and receive assistance in understanding how to effectively address ethical concerns.

The following are some suggestions for respectfully addressing a colleague's behaviors through an informal resolution:

- Reflect and develop clarity regarding the specific behavior and potential ethical violation. Be prepared to directly reference the ethical code or workplace code that is in question or may apply. Seeking consultation prior to addressing the behavior is recommended.
- Be mindful of an organization's hierarchy, identify the appropriate person with whom you can discuss your concern, as well as who you can follow up with if your concern is not appropriately addressed (peer, direct supervisor, human resources employee, licensing board).
- Some counselors may be concerned about retaliation if they engage in a form of whistle-blowing, or if they address the behavior of a powerful colleague. In this instance, it is recommended that you seek outside consultation for the best way to proceed.
- Directly and clearly state your concerns about your colleague's behavior as well as expectations for the appropriate way to proceed (asking that your colleague cease to engage in a specific behavior and/or asking her to receive additional guidance on how to rectify the issue, such as training or supervision). You may lack information regarding the behavior and ask for clarification during this discussion.
- Be mindful that confrontations can be anxiety producing, especially those regarding professional ethics, so take steps to mediate the anxiety by focusing on facts in a nonaggressive manner. Remember that the goal is to serve society and the communities in which we work; the focus is on protecting clients and the community by engaging in ethical behaviors. However, an additional goal is to protect your colleague who may be at risk of ethical misconduct.

Of note, APA further states that informal resolutions should take place when "appropriate" and if the resolution does not violate issues of confidentiality. Therefore, counselors must be able not only to work through potential reactions to having to confront colleagues, but also be able to determine if it is an appropriate method to resolve the issue and if there are issues of confidentiality (see Chapter 2). An example would be an unethical behavior by another counselor, as reported by your client. Confidentiality protects your client's statements. Depending on the severity of the violation, such as an inappropriate relationship, methods for proceeding may include informing the client of the options for making a complaint to an ethics board, or offering to make the complaint on the client's behalf if given his or her consent to do so.

In the case when a colleague's unethical behavior seems severe and is not bound by confidentiality, the APA's Standard 1.05, Reporting Ethical Violations, states the following:

*If an apparent ethical violation has substantially harmed or is likely to substantially harm a person or organization and is not appropriate for informal resolution under Standard 1.04, Informal Resolution of Ethical Violations, or is not resolved properly in that fashion, psychologists take further action appropriate to the situation. Such action might include referral to state or national committees on professional ethics, to state licensing boards, or to the appropriate institutional authorities. This standard does not apply when an intervention would violate confidentiality rights or when psychologists have been retained to review the work of another psychologist whose professional conduct is in question. (APA, 2017, p. 4)*

ACA imposes similar standards regarding how to report ethical violations. ACA Standard I.2.b., Reporting Ethical Violations, states the following:

*If an apparent violation has substantially harmed or is likely to substantially harm a person or organization and is not appropriate for informal resolution or is not resolved properly, counselors take further action depending on the situation. Such action may include referral to state or national committees on professional ethics, voluntary national certification bodies, state licensing boards, or appropriate institutional authorities. The confidentiality rights of clients should be considered in all actions. This standard does not apply when counselors have been retained to review the work of another counselor whose professional conduct is in question (e.g., consultation, expert testimony). (ACA, 2014, p. 19)*

In general, counselors may be inclined to "protect" a colleague by choosing an informal resolution or by not following up with a **formal resolution** when a colleague has not corrected unethical behavior. A counselor may avoid "telling" on a colleague based on a variety of factors, some of which were listed earlier. It is important to be aware that both ACA and APA have further ethical standards regarding the responsibility that counselors have to cooperate.

APA Standard 3.09, Cooperation with Other Professionals, states: "When indicated and professionally appropriate, psychologists cooperate with other professionals in order to serve their clients/patients effectively and appropriately" (APA, 2017). Similarly, ACA Standard D.1.b., Forming Relationships, states: "Counselors work to develop and strengthen relationships with colleagues from other disciplines to best serve clients" (ACA, 2014, p. 10). Notice here that neither code is referring to the willful choice to ignore unethical behavior in colleagues.

## ACTIVITY 7.3

Recall a recent incident in which you received feedback from a peer. Identify the following information regarding this incident: What was my initial or "knee jerk" reaction? How did my body respond? What were my thoughts? How did I feel about this? Did this impact my perception of my peer? Did it impact my later interactions with my peer? Was the delivery of the feedback effective? If not, in what way could the feedback have been delivered more effectively?

## VIGNETTES FOR DISCUSSION

### Instructions

Think through the ethical dilemmas represented by the following short vignettes, and answer the questions that follow as honestly as you can. Remember to monitor your reactions, keeping track of any that include shaming the counselor for "bad" behavior or for being a "bad counselor." Focus on internal and external factors that may have led to this behavior. Now is the time to notice if there are any patterns in your reactions, or the substance of your reactions, and to discuss these in supervision and consultation. This is valuable information for your reflection on what some of your personal biases and blind spots may be. (See the Appendix, Typical Cognitive and Emotional Reactions, at the end of this book.)

### Vignette 1

*Louise is working in a community mental health setting, earning hours toward her license. She notices that a fellow counselor has been showing up late to meetings and at least one appointment with a client. One afternoon, she smells alcohol on her colleague as they leave the office. She is not sure if the counselor had just finished a session with a client or was only in the office to complete paperwork. Louise is concerned that her colleague may be experiencing a problem with alcohol, and is also concerned that this may be affecting the colleague's work. She recognizes that this is a change in behavior for her colleague, much different than when they first met earlier this year.*

### Resolving the Ethical Dilemma

Take some time to think through the following questions. Write down your thoughts for each one.

1. What is the dilemma here?
2. What should Louise do?
3. Which codes may apply to this dilemma?

*(continued)*

## VIGNETTES FOR DISCUSSION (continued)

4. Does this require an informal resolution or direct reporting to an ethics board?
5. Should Louise seek consultation?
6. Are there other ethical codes to which she may need to refer to answer this dilemma?

Addressing an ethical dilemma may require counselors to review several ethical codes. For example, if you are working from the ACA Code of Ethics, did you consider the section entitled "C.2.g., Impairment," when you answered question 3? The ACA standard on impairment states:

> Counselors monitor themselves for signs of impairment from their own physical, mental, or emotional problems and refrain from offering or providing professional services when impaired. They seek assistance for problems that reach the level of professional impairment, and, if necessary, they limit, suspend, or terminate their professional responsibilities until it is determined that they may safely resume their work. Counselors assist colleagues or supervisors in recognizing their own professional impairment and provide consultation and assistance when warranted with colleagues or supervisors showing signs of impairment and intervene as appropriate to prevent imminent harm to clients. (ACA, 2014, p. 13)

### Vignette 2

> Ty is working in a group practice with three colleagues. One of his colleagues has been providing individual therapy to a 15-year-old female client, treating her for anxiety over the past 3 months. Treatment has generally focused on reducing anxiety and working through conflicts she is having with her mother. One day, the 15-year-old's mother asked to meet with the colleague to discuss more specific methods for parenting her daughter, as well as ways to assist her daughter with managing her anxiety. Unsure if it is appropriate to have a separate session with the client's mother, the colleague consults with Ty.
>
> Given the client's reported comfort with her mother having a session to discuss parenting techniques and the focus of the session, Ty responds that it appears to be appropriate. One month later, he notices that his colleague is continuing to have individual appointments with the client's mother. When he asks about this, the colleague says, "When she arrived for her appointment to discuss her daughter she began to share that she was experiencing a significant amount of anxiety herself, and so I have been seeing her separately to help her with that."

### Resolving the Ethical Dilemma

Take some time to think through the following questions. Write down your thoughts for each one.

1. Is this an ethical dilemma? If so, what may it be?
2. What should Ty do?
3. Which codes may apply to this dilemma?

*(continued)*

> **VIGNETTES FOR DISCUSSION (*continued*)**
>
> 4. Does this require an informal resolution or direct reporting to the ethics board?
> 5. What are some options for appropriate ways to proceed?
> 6. Should Ty seek consultation?
>
> In addition to reviewing codes directly related to confronting colleagues, you may have to review other codes as they relate to this vignette. For example, here are two codes that appear relevant to this ethical dilemma.
>
> *APA Code 3.05, Multiple Relationships: (a) A multiple relationship occurs when a psychologist is in a professional role with a person and (1) at the same time is in another role with the same person, (2) at the same time is in a relationship with a person closely associated with or related to the person with whom the psychologist has the professional relationship, or (3) promises to enter into another relationship in the future with the person or a person closely associated with or related to the person. A psychologist refrains from entering into a multiple relationship if the multiple relationship could reasonably be expected to impair the psychologist's objectivity, competence, or effectiveness in performing his or her functions as a psychologist, or otherwise risks exploitation or harm to the person with whom the professional relationship exists. Multiple relationships that would not reasonably be expected to cause impairment or risk exploitation or harm are not unethical. . . . (APA, 2017, p. 6)*
>
> *ACA Code B.7.b., Disclosure of Confidential Information: When consulting with colleagues, counselors do not disclose confidential information that reasonably could lead to the identification of a client or other person or organization with whom they have a confidential relationship unless they have obtained the prior consent of the person or organization or the disclosure cannot be avoided. They disclose information only to the extent necessary to achieve the purposes of the consultation. (ACA, 2014, p. 8)*

## Dilemma 2: Sticky Situation—What Do I Do If My Workplace Rules Seem to Contradict My Code of Ethics?

There will be times throughout your career when work policies or procedures will seem to be at odds with your ethical obligations. A popular dilemma arises when working with insurance companies that will only cover a certain number of sessions, or will only provide reimbursement if the client is given a specific diagnosis. Counselors often grapple with the reality of needing to be honest with insurance and available to provide care for their clients. In this situation, counselors may struggle with wanting to withhold information from, or provide false information to, an insurance company. However, falsifying insurance information is unethical and an ethical violation.

Outside of issues with insurance, certain workplaces create almost immediate conflicts with either the APA or ACA codes of ethics, specifically with regard to confidentiality. Correctional environments often employ counselors, creating a situation in which the jail or prison itself is the client, as opposed to the inmates who the counselor is treating. As noted in Chapter 2, whereas the practice of psychology focuses on respecting clients' privacy and confidentiality, many areas of forensic and correctional psychology focus on the protection of society, or the legal client, which is not necessarily the client with whom the counselor meets and may in fact be an institution, a lawyer, or a representative of the court. In this instance, counselors are often confronted with the realities of their clients possessing limited rights and confidentiality, as the institution, or legal client, is privy to some, or all, of their information.

Additionally, given the physical environment in which services are provided in some of these situations, maintaining confidentiality can be nearly impossible. For example, counselors working in prisons may provide services on a housing unit where other inmates see that a prisoner is engaging in contact with mental health staff. Concerns regarding confidentiality have also been noted regarding counselors who work within the military system, understanding that areas specific to "fitness of duty" may be accessible to or reported to military administrators (Prosek & Holm, 2014). Accordingly, it is necessary for the counselor to take as many "reasonable" steps as possible to navigate this sticky situation and uphold the profession's ethical standards.

APA Standard 1.03, Conflicts Between Ethics and Organizational Demands, states the following regarding **organization conflicts** between a counselor's workplace and ethical responsibilities:

> *If the demands of an organization with which psychologists are affiliated or for whom they are working are in conflict with this Ethics Code, psychologists clarify the nature of the conflict, make known their commitment to the Ethics Code, and take reasonable steps to resolve the conflict consistent with the General Principles and Ethical Standards of the Ethics Code. Under no circumstances may this standard be used to justify or defend violating human rights. (APA, 2017, p. 4)*

ACA has similar guidelines regarding this conflict, as stated in I.2.d., Organizational Conflicts:

> *If the demands of an organization with which counselors are affiliated pose a conflict with the* ACA Code of Ethics, *counselors specify the nature of such conflicts and express to their supervisors or other responsible officials their commitment to the* ACA Code of Ethics *and, when possible, work through the appropriate channels to address the situation. (ACA, 2014, p. 19)*

**ORGANIZATION CONFLICTS** - Situations that arise when an organization or workplace has policies that conflict with a counselor's ethical standards.

## VIGNETTE FOR DISCUSSION

### Instructions

As before, think through the ethical dilemmas represented by the following short vignette, and answer the questions that follow as honestly as you can.

### Vignette 3

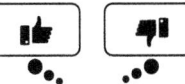

*Gordon works in a substance abuse program as a group counselor. One of the rules of the program is that clients must remain abstinent. If they do not, counselors may have to report clients' actions to their parole officers, they may no longer be provided with Suboxone, or they may eventually be discharged from the program. During a group therapy session, a client informs Gordon that he relapsed on heroin over the weekend. Gordon is concerned that sharing this information with the client's parole officer or the substance abuse program may lead to consequences that will negatively impact the client's treatment, as well as their therapeutic relationship. He feels unsure of how to proceed and consults with a colleague. The colleague informs Gordon that she rarely reports her clients' relapses to parole or to the program despite the rule, citing confidentiality and the need to protect the therapeutic relationship.*

### Resolving the Ethical Dilemma

Take some time to think through the following questions. Write down your thoughts for each one.

1. What is the ethical dilemma?
2. Which codes may apply to this dilemma?
3. What are some options for appropriate ways to proceed?
4. Does this require an informal resolution or direct reporting to the ethics board?

In this case, we see an ethical dilemma related to workplace rules and confidentiality. To inform a sound ethical decision, the counselor will need to refer to the ethical standards and sections listed in this chapter, but also to Chapter 2 related to confidentiality. Standards regarding informed consent are important to review. There are also other ethical codes that may be relevant. For example, the APA's Standard 1.03, Conflicts Between Ethics and Organizational Demand, states that

> if the demands of an organization with which psychologists are affiliated or for whom they are working are in conflict with this Ethics Code, psychologists clarify the nature of the conflict, make known their commitment to the Ethics Code and take reasonable steps to resolve the conflict consistent with the General Principles and Ethical Standards of the Ethics Code. Under no circumstances may this standard be used to justify or defend violating human rights. (APA, 2017)

The counselor should also refer to ACA Standard 1.2.d., Organizational Conflicts:

> *If the demands of an organization with which counselors are affiliated pose a conflict with the ACA Code of Ethics, counselors specify the nature of such conflicts and express to their supervisors or other responsible officials their commitment to the ACA Code of Ethics and, when possible, work through the appropriate channels to address the situation.* (ACA, 2014, p. 19)

What other information should be gathered? Did you notice the need to refer to codes regarding informed consent?

# Dilemma 3: What Do I Do if a Supervisor or Someone in a Leadership Position Is Behaving Unethically?

### VIGNETTE FOR DISCUSSION

Again, think through the ethical dilemmas represented by the following short vignette, and answer the questions that follow as honestly as you can.

### Vignette 4

*Ella is working at the Department of Veterans Affairs as a psychology intern, earning hours toward her license. She meets with her direct supervisor on a weekly basis for individual and also group supervision with other interns. Last week, as she was leaving work, she noticed her supervisor kissing a client in the parking lot. She is aware that this person is a client of the VA because she has seen the person arriving for appointments over the past few months.*

### Resolving the Ethical Dilemma

Take some time to think through the following questions. Write down your thoughts for each one.

1. What is the ethical dilemma in this vignette?
2. Which codes may apply to this dilemma?
3. What are some options for appropriate ways to proceed?
4. Which codes may apply to this dilemma?
5. Does this require an informal resolution or direct reporting to the ethics board?
6. What aspects of the therapist's personality or experience may make it particularly challenging for her to address an authority figure's behavior?

In this case it may not feel appropriate or safe to approach the supervisor directly. The following standards apply to this example:

> *ACA Standard I.2.c., Consultation:* When uncertain about whether a particular situation or course of action may be in violation of the ACA Code of Ethics, counselors consult with other counselors who are knowledgeable about ethics and the ACA Code of Ethics, with colleagues, or with appropriate authorities, such as the ACA Ethics and Professional Standards Department. *(ACA, 2014, p. 19)*

> *APA Standard 10.05, Sexual Intimacies with Current Therapy Clients/Patients:* Psychologists do not engage in sexual intimacies with current therapy clients/patients. *(APA, 2017, p. 15)*

> *ACA Standard A.5.a., Sexual and/or Romantic Relationships Prohibited:* Sexual and/or romantic counselor–client interactions or relationships with current clients, their romantic partners, or their family members are prohibited. This prohibition applies to both in-person and electronic interactions or relationships. *(ACA, 2014, p. 5)*

## CASE STUDY VIGNETTE

### Instructions

Following the case study vignette, consider the questions on how to make an ethical decision to resolve this dilemma. Again, remember to monitor your reactions, keeping track of any that include shaming the counselor for "bad" behavior or for being a "bad counselor." Focus on the internal and external factors that may have led to this behavior. Now is the time to notice if there are any patterns in your reactions, or the substance of your reactions, and to discuss these in supervision and consultation. This is valuable information for your reflection on what some of your personal biases and blind spots may be. (See the Appendix, Typical Cognitive and Emotional Reactions, at the end of this book.)

### Case Study

*Tim is working in a prison where he provides individual and group therapy to incarcerated men. He works with several other psychologists, counselors, and social workers. Often, multiple mental health professionals interact with the same clients through individual therapy, group therapy, or some other form of assessment. Tim has one direct supervisor within the prison and an administrator who oversees multiple prisons.*

*Tim has been working biweekly in individual therapy with Robert, a young man who was diagnosed with bipolar disorder. Tim has been providing Robert with psycho-education about his condition, monitoring any changes in his mood or functioning, and assisting him in developing stress-reducing techniques. Robert has a history of substance abuse, so he also attends group therapy with one of Tim's colleagues on a weekly basis. Robert reported some dissatisfaction with this group in the past but has continued, partly based on Tim's encouragement to work through*

*(continued)*

## CASE STUDY VIGNETTE (continued)

*issues related to his recovery. They seem to have a positive working relationship, and both believe that Robert is making progress toward his goals.*

*Two days ago, Tim was speaking with Dan, a colleague who has been facilitating Robert's substance abuse–focused therapy group. Dan commented, "I don't think it's worth our time to see Robert, he's a manipulator and nothing but a criminal." Tim was surprised by Dan's comments and asked him to clarify his concerns. Dan did not provide any behavioral examples or history to support his claims that Robert was a "manipulator"; rather, he stated that he did not like Robert and was generally uninterested in providing his treatment.*

*Concerned about this interaction, Tim approaches his direct supervisor and discusses the conversation he had with Dan. His supervisor does not share Tim's concerns, stating, "Maybe he's right. It's going to be the case that most of these guys here are full of it." Tim attempts to voice another concern regarding the quality of Dan's care if he is not invested in assisting his clients. His supervisor comments, "It doesn't really matter if they are all helped, we just need to have at least 10 people in a room to justify our staff numbers. Don't worry about it."*

*Tim is now left feeling anxious and frustrated that some of the counselors do not appear to be invested in helping all the clients. He also begins to wonder if he was wrong when perceiving Robert's sincerity about participating in treatment.*

### Resolving the Ethical Dilemma

Think about the following questions. Write your answers down before moving on to the discussion.

1. What are the ethical dilemmas in this case?
2. Should Tim actively address this situation? What are the options for doing so?
3. Should he gather more information? If so, what?
4. Based on a review of the APA Ethics Code and the ACA Codes of Ethics, which code(s) should Tim rely on to resolve this dilemma?
5. As you review the situation, should Tim engage in an informal or a formal resolution? How should he go about this?

### Case Study Discussion Questions

1. What information does Tim still need to gather in order to better understand the dilemma?
2. Which variables within this vignette are important to note in order to best understand this situation?
3. Which gray areas were presented in this case, but not discussed, that could raise additional ethical dilemmas?
4. To the individuals mentioned in this vignette, assign different sex, gender, sexual orientation, culture, socioeconomic, nation of origin,

*(continued)*

### CASE STUDY VIGNETTE (continued)

immigrant status, refugee status, primary language spoken, disability, or other variables. Would any of these variables impact your perception of the statements or actions within this vignette? If so, how? If not, what leads you to believe that none of these variables would impact your thinking or reactions? This information regarding your beliefs and reactions would be useful to discuss going forward in supervision.

## CHAPTER DISCUSSION QUESTIONS

1. What do I need to be aware of with regard to myself and my workplace in order to remain open to confronting colleagues?
2. What steps would you follow if you encountered a sticky situation in the future? If you know of a sticky situation currently, what can you do now to minimize its impact?
3. How can I best integrate my ethical guidelines when working in workplace settings that either follow a separate set of ethical standards (e.g., ACA vs. APA) or different standards of practice?

### ACTIVITY 7.4

It is important to understand exactly what is expected of us. Investigate ethical and state standards regarding reporting unethical behavior, as well as any rules put forth by your place of work (see Chapter 1 on gathering information in your state).

Write these down and discuss them with your supervisors or instructors to compare and review. Then, identify and write down exactly how you would personally report unethical behavior at the state level.

It is also important that counselors know the resources that are available to them. Think through the following. Writing these down will also be helpful to have as a resource.

- Do you belong to a professional organization that offers resources, such as someone to call, in order to sort out ethical dilemmas? Do you know what those resources are? If you belong to an organization, but you are unsure of its capabilities in this regard, investigate this. If you do not belong to a professional organization, now is the time to join.

- Within your workplace, is there a resource that you can reach out to regarding concerns with your leadership? Investigate the protocol for reporting unethical behavior by a supervisor or someone in a leadership position.

- Establish an explicit agreement with your colleagues that you wish to be directly informed if they are ever concerned that you may be engaging in unethical behavior and that they are open to being informed if they do the same.

# CONCLUSION

As explored in this chapter, holding our colleagues accountable and informing them of apparent ethical violations is one of our duties as professional counselors. Given the actions of our colleagues, we may engage in informal or formal resolutions. Variables that may impact our response to observing ethical dilemmas may include the power structure of an organization or power dynamics within a relationship. Counselors are also responsible for acknowledging any potential conflicts between workplace rules and ethical standards, and addressing them accordingly.

## PERSONAL INVENTORY: QUESTIONS FOR FURTHER EXPLORATION

### PROFESSIONAL EXPERIENCES

1. Have you had an experience in the past in which your boss, manager, or professional superior seemed to behave inappropriately? What was your reaction and response to this?
2. Have you had an experience at work or school in which you noticed policies or procedures that seemed to be in violation of either ethical standards or rules? What was your reaction and how did you respond?

### PERSONAL EXPERIENCES

1. Can you recall messages that you have received throughout your life regarding the appropriate way to respond when you noticed inappropriate behavior? Reflect on messages you have received through your family of origin, your culture, and your training.
2. Do you remember a time in the past when you felt a role conflict, such as struggling to maintain two separate but seemingly incompatible roles? What was your experience of this and how did you respond?

# REFERENCES

American Counseling Association. (2014). *2014 ACA code of ethics*. Retrieved from https://www.counseling.org/resources/aca-code-of-ethics.pdf

American Psychological Association. (2017). *Ethical principles of psychologists and code of conduct* (2002, amended June 1, 2010 and January 1, 2017). Retrieved from http://www.apa.org/ethics/code/index.aspx

Brennan, C. (2013). Ensuring ethical practice: Guidelines for mental health counselors in private practice. *Journal of Mental Health Counseling, 35*, 245–261.

Furr, S., & Brown-Rice, K. (2016). Doctoral students' knowledge of educators' problems of professional competency. *Training and Education in Professional Psychology, 10,* 223–230. doi:10.1037/tep0000131

Gladding, S. (2013). *Counseling: A comprehensive profession* (7th ed.). New York, NY: Pearson.

Herlihy, B., & Dufrene, R. (2011). Current and emerging ethical issues in counseling: A Delphi study of expert opinions. *Counseling and Values, 56,* 1–15.

Olson, S., Brown-Rice, K., & Keller, N. (2016). Mental health practitioners' knowledge of colleague problems of professional competency. *Journal of Mental Health Counseling, 38,* 308–326. doi:10.17744/mehc.38.4.03

Prosek, E., & Holm, J. (2014). Counselors and the military: When protocol and ethics conflict. *The Professional Counselor, 4,* 93–102.

Remley, T., & Herlihy, B. (2014). *Ethical, legal, and professional issues in counseling* (4th ed.). New York, NY: Pearson.

Rice, A. (2015). Using scholarship on whistleblowing to inform peer ethics reporting. *Professional Psychology: Research and Practice, 46,* 298–305. doi:10.1037/pro0000038

# PART IV  RECOMMENDATIONS

# CHAPTER 8

# SELF-CARE

Counselors are members of a noble profession. We engage in rigorous study and training in order to assist others with living improved lives. Our research, education, and treatment are driven by high principles such as beneficence, integrity, and justice. Most of us enter into this field because we wish to help. We are helping professionals who are trained to put the needs of our clients first, to consider their vulnerabilities and work to protect them, to recognize areas of weakness and provide skills for increasing areas of strength. We aim to improve clients' quality of life despite any presence of mental illness or environmental stress. We should be proud of our choice to become counselors, and we receive many benefits from doing so. We will have the privilege of knowing many clients and colleagues throughout our careers and will experience our own personal growth as a result of some of our professional experiences. With this gift comes great responsibility, and one of our responsibilities is to remain healthy so that we may provide excellent service to those with whom we work.

This type of work can be a challenge. At times, it will challenge our patience and conviction. During difficult times, it may challenge our basic understanding of others, the world, and of ourselves. Counselors work within many challenging environments: within hospitals, within prisons, in emergency situations; with those who are ill, those who are violent, those who are disadvantaged, and those who, for a variety of reasons, may show little improvement despite receiving help. Datillo (2015) stated:

> *Next to air traffic controllers, police officers, firefighters, and professional bomb squad units, mental health professionals have one of the most stressful professions in the world. By the very nature of the work that we do, we repeatedly deal with psychologically toxic situations in which we are often expected to assist individuals who are suffering from some of the most arduous and complex disorders found within the broad spectrum of mental illness.* (p. 393)

In order to remain healthy, despite stress-inducing situations and work environments, we must take care of ourselves. Taking care of ourselves as helping professionals may be one of the wisest choices we make throughout our careers, for ourselves and for those with whom we work.

This chapter will use a different format from others in this textbook. We will cover what constitutes self-care, why it is necessary for engaging in ethical behavior, and what may impact our functioning over time. Terms such as *burnout, compassion fatigue,* and *vicarious trauma* will be discussed, and we will offer recommendations for ways to manage stress and maintain excellence in our work. We will review multiple vignettes that describe a variety of counselors' responses to their work in order to provide practice with evaluating aspects of their functioning as well as ways that they could improve.

## NEED FOR SELF-CARE

Corey (2013) stated, "Ethical decision making is an evolutionary process that requires you to be continually open and self-reflective" (p. 51). Self-reflection is a tool that counselors can use, but it is one that must be cultivated, welcomed, practiced on a regular basis, and supported by effective counselor **self-care**. Engaging in effective and consistent self-care allows counselors to maintain excellence in work and a healthy balance in their lives. Although self-care is essential for counselors' health, as well as their ethical behavior, training programs may not properly include education and assistance with developing a self-care routine (Bamonti et al., 2014). Given the trend to not recommend therapy for students in graduate programs, the need for teaching and practicing self-care, as a core competency, has become even more essential.

Colman et al. (2016) examined if self-care practiced by graduate students produced any significant changes or results in their functioning. They found gains in self-compassion, decreased psychological distress, and improved life satisfaction. Wise, Hersh, and Gibson (2012) described principles of self-care as including: "an emphasis on flourishing," intentionality, awareness of reciprocity in care of self and others, and the benefits of integrating self-care into daily practices or as a routine, rather than an add-on activity.

Engaging in the active and dynamic process of self-care is the pathway toward consistent ethical behavior. Counselors rely on themselves as the tool by which they provide services. For this reason, counselors are at risk of becoming depleted in a variety of ways. Our functioning immediately impacts our work. Counselors who have not taken care of themselves become vulnerable to losing their effectiveness at best, and at worst may be at risk of unethical behavior. In this chapter, we review these dilemmas and walk through how the American Psychological Association's Ethical Principles of Psychologists and Code of Conduct and the American Counseling Association's Code of Ethics address the need for self-care.

> **SELF-CARE** - A dynamic and continuous process that includes attending to multiple aspects of the counselor's health and functioning (see Figure 8.1).

## HOW CAN COUNSELORS ENGAGE IN SELF-CARE?

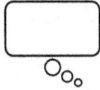

Self-care has been thought about and discussed for some time. However, there is a shortage of research into effective types of self-care, as well as specific counselor needs based on environmental or work conditions. Notwithstanding, most counselors will be encouraged to engage in self-care, and many will try to engage in some form thereof. Turner et al. (2005) surveyed psychology interns and found that common self-care activities included social support from family and friends, seeking pleasurable experiences, and humor. Self-care can be taught, as a skill and as a practice, and is a practice that should begin during internships (Testa & Sangganjanavanich, 2015). The importance and practice of self-care, however, could—and should—begin within educational or school environments to establish a base level of knowledge regarding the necessity of self-care, as well as potential strategies and tools for managing reactions to counseling work.

As a field, we acknowledge our ethical obligation to maintain health and effectiveness and often focus on specific methods for doing so. Historically, when graduate students were required to participate in therapy, it served the purpose of assisting students with personal growth and development while allowing them the experience of "being on the other side of the couch." Today, many, if not most, programs do not require that their students participate in therapy. Rather, it is recommended. Given our personalities and internal motivations, we are all responsive to, and triggered by, individual situations and interpersonal factors. The best method for determining what is motivating us and what our needs are is to engage in therapy. Regarding group counselors, Corey (2013) stated, "I believe that extensive self-exploration is necessary for trainees to identify countertransference feelings, to recognize blind spots and biases, and to use their personal attributes effectively in their group work" (p. 63). It will be a challenge, if indeed it is possible at all, to be fully aware of our reactions to clients without receiving assistance through counseling or clinical supervision.

Burkholder and Burkholder (2014) surveyed counseling faculty members' understanding of their students' ethical misconduct as well their beliefs regarding methods for ways to prevent ethical misconduct. Regarding preventative methods, faculty members identified education and training, gatekeeping and screening, monitoring, personal growth, and support. We argue that personal growth is a necessary aspect of engaging in ethical behavior, is best accomplished through engagement in therapy, and is best maintained through additional therapy as well as other support methods discussed in this chapter. Given that therapy is an intimately personal experience, it will be important to find a counselor or psychologist who is competent in understanding your unique cultural experiences, as well as your personal background and needs.

## Elements of Self-Care

Self-care for counselors is a professional responsibility that includes more than eating healthy, going to the gym, spending time with friends, and using humor as a coping skill. Although all of these activities are helpful, they are not enough to maintain a counselor's health and well-being given the nature of this work. Self-care for counselors should include physical health, social health, personal therapy, supervision or consultation, an understanding of personal and professional meaning, identification and negotiation of personal narratives, and environmental or workplace variables that support personal and professional health. Each of these factors

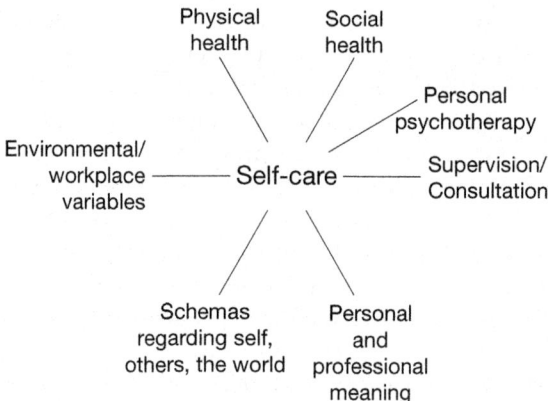

**FIGURE 8.1** A self-care model for counselors.

may be more or less influential or needed given the specific counselor and her or his context (Figure 8.1).

## Physical Health

Physical activity may help with preventing burnout (Gerber et al., 2015). However, more generally, counselors' physical health can have an immediate impact on their work as well as their overall functioning. *Health* is a broad term and there should be no assumptions that a counselor must be physically healthy in order to be effective. With regard to physical health as it applies to self-care, we assert that it should be regularly considered, respected, and prioritized.

Self-care recommendations have long included exercise, eating well, and engaging in practices that promote physical heath. In addition to these, it is important to note that counselors should consider the impact of their work on their physical health—from the physical conditions of the workplace (the types of chairs that counselors sit in, if there are windows, if food is available) to the impact of stress on the body. For counselors who work in locked facilities, such as prisons or psychiatric hospitals, entry and exit may be difficult, and limit access to sunlight or fresh air. Counselors may need to make accommodations in their work routines in order to best support their physical health and well-being.

## Social Health

A wise colleague once said: "Your home life should be much larger in comparison to your work life." Through this statement, she was explaining the need to have fulfilling relationships and experiences outside of work in order to avoid "getting our needs met" *through* our work. As we are social beings, the health of our relationships has an immediate impact on our functioning.

Given the fact that counselors may be spending many hours, throughout their days and weeks, interacting with many different people, it is possible to wish to spend some time alone once there is an opportunity to do so. Isolation, particularly during stressful times, may be rewarding but at the same time may not leave a counselor refreshed or prepared for work. Isolation can also have a personal impact. Whereas every counselor differs in terms of the need for socialization, the quality of it should be healthy, regardless of the amount of socialization that counselors engage in. Also, if the majority of a counselor's social interactions are occurring through work, the counselor's work–life balance may be skewed.

Social health also includes healthy relationships built on acceptance of differences, inclusion of diverse backgrounds, and sociopolitical realities. Underrepresented counselors (e.g., based on race, ethnicity nationality, gender, citizenship status, etc.), as well as other marginalized groups, may be faced with stressful work conditions, tense interactions with colleagues, and nuanced client–therapist interactions based on the groups of which the counselor is perceived to be a part. Engaging with friends, community members, peers, colleagues, and supervisors who understand the sociopolitical realities of marginalized communities, and understanding how issues of racism, sexism, microaggressions, homophobia, and other forms of oppression impact the function and well-being of counselors is not only important, but in fact critical to self-care and well-being.

Having new and inspiring experiences with others can also support overall social health. Similarly, if a personal relationship is unhealthy or feels "draining," it is important to remain mindful of how it may be impacting other areas of functioning. In the case where a counselor has relational concerns, supervision or consultation can be helpful for identifying if this is impacting how a counselor perceives or relates to clients, particularly given that therapy occurs in the context of a relationship. These types of issues may be best understood by receiving assistance, as our ability to remain objective may at times be compromised.

## Personal Therapy

The choice to engage in therapy is a personal one. We also participate in therapy for a variety of reasons. Given the nature of our work, it would be wise to engage in therapy during early career stages to have the experience of being the client, as well the opportunity to work through any personal issues or blind spots. Choosing a mental health provider with whom you are comfortable is crucial, as any benefits are reliant on a counseling relationship that is built on safety and trust.

We assert that having a strong understanding of one's own internal dynamics is important for developing self-awareness and an ability to exercise judgment with regard to ethical dilemmas. Taking care of our own mental health is a requirement for doing good work; there is no self-care absent our mental health. Likewise, and similar to our physical health, it is important to regularly monitor how our work may be impacting our mental health and well-being.

## Supervision and Consultation

Supervision is required throughout training and prelicensure, and often for furthering development of particular skill sets or areas of expertise. Part of professional development involves learning how to effectively engage in supervision. Supervisors are often in a position of authority during a counselor's training experiences, and therefore counselors may feel apprehensive about being open and vulnerable. However, it is the counselor's responsibility to participate in this process. If there are specific variables that are preventing a counselor from feeling comfortable with a supervisor, it is important to address these as best as possible. Given that the quality of the supervisory relationship may impact a supervisee's willingness to self-disclose, it is recommended that supervisees become educated regarding how to effectively use supervision (Sweeney & Creaner, 2014). Supervision is a process that should continue throughout our careers. There are supervisors available in private practice postlicensure, as well as opportunities for focused training.

In addition to individual or group supervision, there are also consultation groups or go-to colleagues with whom to consult. Engaging in consultation regarding counseling practices ought to be frequent. Through this engagement, counselors are able to feel a sense of connection and community, and consultation also serves as a useful source for better understanding how to respond to ethical situations. As to whom a counselor engages with in consultation, it is best to find colleagues outside of friend networks and who are comfortable remaining objective and directive when needed. Consultations are also most effective when the atmosphere is safe for others to provide honest feedback. This is one way of engaging in checks and balances and keeping ourselves grounded (see Chapter 7, Confronting Colleagues and Other Sticky Situations).

## Personal and Professional Meaning

Having an understanding of the purpose or meaning behind our daily lives and our careers is important for avoiding burnout and other negative reactions to challenging work. Personal and professional meaning can be threatened by this type of work. When counselors find meaning *through* their work, such as "I am here to help others," then experiencing treatment failures, or other work-related disappointments, may challenge their purpose. It is important to identify and repeatedly return to the underlying purpose—one that is not contingent upon results or external factors.

Questions such as "why am I here?" and "what is the point?" should be examined regularly, as the answers will likely impact the counselor's ability to remain resilient and intentional in his or her actions.

## Schemas Regarding the Self, Others, and the World

Our experiences impact our schemas, which can be understood as our worldviews that directly impact our reactions to others, our perceptions of events, and our judgments about good vs. bad behaviors, thoughts, and emotions. Clues about our schemas are the thoughts that we experience or generate throughout each day. If we notice that we are having cynical thoughts, they may be reflecting deeper views. For example, many developing counselors feel disheartened when they realize that some clients fail to tell the truth or engage in what appears to be manipulative behavior. They may begin to think that clients should not be trusted. A series of these thoughts may indicate a change in the counselors' schemas about counseling work that may impact their ability to accurately perceive and respond to clients' presentations or needs.

Counselors within forensic settings may frequently experience what could be considered boundary violations by their clients (boundaries in this case not referring to breaking ethical boundaries, but rather boundaries of the rules of relationships). It was found that the frequency and impact of these violations toward the counselor were related to higher rates of depersonalization, also possibly leading to cynical attitudes and feelings toward clients (Johnson, Worthington, Gredecki, & Wilks-Riley, 2016). We are responsible for recognizing factors, conditions, and circumstances that cause negative beliefs and reactions, and challenging them in order to maintain our health, effectiveness, and ethical judgment.

## Environmental and Workplace Variables

We are responsible for identifying and addressing workplace variables that are impacting our effectiveness as counselors. These contextual variables have an immediate impact on our functioning. Even when we may not be able to change them, we must be aware of them so that they do not impede our ability to accurately perceive and respond to ethical dilemmas. These may include workplace norms (see Chapter 3, Professional Boundaries) as well as workplace practices and toxic work conditions that marginalize people based on their social-cultural identities (see Chapter 5, Culturally Competent Treatment).

For example, counselors within a correctional setting may feel pressure to "deal with" an enormous number of emotionally charged and challenging situational variables that come with the territory of working inside a prison or jail. That pressure, explicitly or implicitly stated, could impact a counselor's openness to acknowledging negative reactions to the work. Lack of openness could then affect the counselor's functioning in a variety of ways. In another example, some workplaces include high caseloads and heavy work demands. Counselors within such settings may feel pressure to cope with the pressures without opportunities for immediate support. That could also impact counselors' functioning by reducing their ability to acknowledge their reactions as well as their clients' needs. In cases where workplace environments and practices are oppressive to marginalized communities, counselors may feel unsafe, unsupported, or disengaged. This could impact both the mental health of the counselor and her or his ability to remain present enough to effectively navigate ethical dilemmas.

In cases where the counselor cannot change workplace variables, or when power dynamics are at play, counselors must be mindful of the impact on their ability to be effective and possibly impede their ability to respond appropriately to ethical dilemmas when they arise. Self-care in these instances is critical for maintaining sound clinical and ethical judgment.

# BURNOUT, COMPASSION FATIGUE, AND VICARIOUS TRAUMA

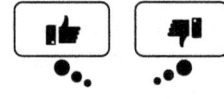

Among disaster responders, it was found that pre-disaster life events, such as personal trauma or psychiatric history, increased risk for mental health problems after disasters (Brooks, Dunn, Amlôt, Greenberg, & Rubin, 2016). Knowing this, it is important to acknowledge what some of our vulnerabilities may be and actively address them in therapy or supervision. As every counselor is unique, every counselor will have a unique response to clients and work conditions. There should be no expectation of how one should or should not respond, just that there will be a response and the best way to manage it is to acknowledge it. Here we review burnout, compassion fatigue, and vicarious trauma as experiences that may impact well-being and ethical decision making.

## Burnout

Burnout has been described as a prolonged response to work-related stress. Burnout can be experienced by anyone at any time, regardless of their profession or their circumstances. Burnout can result in exhaustion, anxiety, insomnia, forgetfulness, changes in eating or sleeping, and diminished feelings of self-efficacy (Matula, 2013). People who are burned out often experience a drastic reduction in energy or motivation. Burnout is associated with a depressive cognitive style as well as cynicism (Bianchi & Schonfeld, 2015; Wei, Wang, & MacDonald, 2015). Similarities between job burnout and depression have been examined and found to have overlapping characteristics (Toker & Biron, 2012).

Although burnout can occur in a variety of situations, specific environments or client populations may lead to unique burnout experiences. In essence, counselors experience burnout differently and certain environments may put us at an increased risk. For example, Lee et al. (2010) found that sex offender and abuse survivor therapists have more emotional disturbances and social difficulties with significant others when compared to other mental health professionals.

## Compassion Fatigue

The concept of compassion fatigue was developed to describe the experience of caregivers. Coined by Joinson (1992), it is different from burnout in that burnout can theoretically happen in any setting, whereas compassion fatigue is specific to caregiving professions. Joinson described the condition as involving overwhelming stress that reduces one's ability to function, leading to apathy and possibly depression. In counseling, it may be used to describe the experience of losing compassion, or having a negative reaction to the counseling work. We may notice colleagues who seem to "not care" or who are "jaded." When we do, we are likely describing someone's experience with compassion fatigue. Those who are empathetic or caring may absorb some of the traumatic stress that their clients are experiencing (Najjar, Davis, Beck-Coon, & Doebbeling, 2009). We can see here that a skill such as empathy may leave us vulnerable to experiencing intense reactions to clients and their stories. Compassion fatigue may also be related to a reduction in the connection or empathy experienced by the counselor. Detachment, however, is not a protective factor. Detachment or being "shut down" is a natural response to feeling cognitively or emotionally overwhelmed, but it is not helpful for the therapeutic process. Rather, a lack of "personal survival strategies" may lead to experiences of compassion fatigue (Huggard, 2003, p. 164).

## Vicarious Traumatization

*Vicarious traumatization* is "the transformation that occurs within the therapist (or other trauma worker) as a result of empathic engagement with the clients' trauma experience and their sequelae" (Pearlman & Mac Ian, 1995, p. 1). Vicarious trauma is understood to transform the counselor's inner experience, as well as his or her experiences of others and the world. This can occur when a counselor is witness to a client's graphic descriptions of trauma, including, but not limited to, sexual abuse or other childhood abuse, sexual assault, experiences with military combat or other war-related experiences, experiences with violence, and experiences with natural disasters or other catastrophes. Vicarious trauma can lead to intrusive thoughts as well as bodily reactions. For example, a counselor who provides intensive trauma-focused therapy for a veteran who experienced loss in combat from gunfire may have an immediate visceral reaction to sounds of gunfire or similar-sounding noises.

Attempts have been made both to understand the causes of vicarious trauma and to develop methods for preventing it. Harrison and Westwood (2009) conducted a qualitative study to identify protective practices against vicarious trauma in mental health professionals. Along with noting that educators, employers, professional bodies, and individual practitioners have a responsibility to address the issue of vicarious trauma, they also concluded that there were several protective factors: countering isolation, developing mindful self-awareness, consciously expanding perspectives to embrace complexity, active optimism, holistic self-care, maintaining clear boundaries, empathy, professional satisfaction, and creating meaning.

## Self-Care Leads to Self-Awareness, Which Leads to Effective Treatment and Ethical Judgment

The previous explanation of the causes of vicarious trauma (i.e., empathetic engagement with clients' trauma) may leave the impression that connecting with those who have experienced trauma can have a negative effect on the counselor. To the contrary, Harrison and Westwood (2009) stated:

> [W]hen clinicians maintain clarity about interpersonal boundaries, when they are able to get very close without fusing or confusing the client's story, experiences, and perspective with their own, this exquisite kind of empathic

> *attunement is nourishing for the therapist and client alike, in part because the therapists recognize it is beneficial to the client. (p. 213)*

This is the crux of the purpose for self-care. Self-care allows effective self-awareness, which in turn allows counselors to know their boundaries and maintain an openness to fully engage with clients. Self-awareness, which is an ongoing process, assists us with identifying our schemas as well as our daily reactions to our work. Corey (2013) stated, "Ethical decision making is an evolutionary process that requires you to be continually open and self-reflective" (p. 51). Self-reflection is a tool that we can use, but it is one that must be cultivated, welcomed, practiced on a regular basis, and supported by effective counselor self-care.

Self-care is not only an effort to reduce stress and improve positive experiences. Rather, on a quest toward true self-care, we must confront aspects of our and our clients' experiences that produce anxiety. These can be related to aspects of our clients' personalities or presenting problems that trigger us. These can also be related to aspects of our own personalities or life experiences, irrespective of our client's presenting problems. Therefore, a central aspect of self-care is self-awareness and critical self-reflection. This quest toward better self-awareness may result in some distress as we confront our worldviews or other aspects of ourselves. This will present an opportunity to benefit from support through supervision or other means.

## Self-Awareness of Socially Constructed Power and Privilege

One of the greatest challenges in self-awareness and critical self-reflection is acknowledging aspects of our identities that have been given socially constructed power and privilege. As noted in Chapter 5, there are groups that historically have been given power and privilege by virtue of being born into these groups (e.g., White, heterosexual, male, affluent).

Self-awareness around aspects of ourselves that have these socially constructed privileges is essential for managing our reactions and for providing appropriate treatment. Given what we believe is valid mistrust and hesitation in working with counselors who represent groups with socially constructed power, counselors must engage in continuous self-reflection on the role of power and privilege in their work, in the therapeutic relationship, in treatment planning and diagnosis.

One of the premises we have underscored throughout the book is our belief that no counselor wants to intentionally hurt others or engage in unethical behaviors. However, lack of self-awareness about power dynamics is one of the areas in which we have the potential to oppress, stigmatize, or marginalize others. It is our ethical duty to be aware of our biases, assumptions, and prejudice. Yet, as scholars note, this is not an easy task.

For example, in a qualitative study of White individuals committed to combating racism, the authors found that participants experienced various challenges (Smith & Redington, 2010). A commonly reported challenge was related to "interpersonal conflicts." White participants reported that both their personal and public relationships were affected when they engaged in racial advocacy. The study highlighted the importance of ongoing critical self-reflection. Given that identities that have been granted socially constructed power often operate as a "norm," biases and assumptions usually operate at a subconscious level. In their study, one participant noted that regardless of the commitment to fighting racism, "I still forget I'm White" (p. 564).

Historical and current events of discrimination have created feelings of mistrust and discomfort by clients from marginalized populations (Shim, Compton, Rust, Druss, & Kaslow, 2009) when they are in treatment by counselors who resemble people who have historically oppressed others (e.g., male, White, heterosexual). Studies that examine the perception of counselors, for example, show that African American clients perceive therapists as being older, male, and White—and thus as being aloof, uncaring, or out of touch with the lived experiences of African American communities and so unable to provide relevant treatment (Thompson, Bazile, & Akbar, 2004). Perceived discrimination based on sexism and racism has also been found among lesbian, gay, bisexual, and transgender (LGBT) racial/ethnic minorities, who may mistrust counselors due to discrimination and mistreatment of both racial/ethnic minorities and gender-nonconforming, lesbian, gay, bisexual, or queer individuals (Nadal, 2013; see Chapter 5).

However, relatively little has been done to help counselors manage issues of power and privilege in the therapy room. As a result, counselors are often left on their own to figure out how to manage both their clients and themselves. Deliberate self-discovery is probably the best method to ensure that counselors do not engage in oppressive or microaggressive acts in therapy (Mazzula & Nadal, 2015). However, this process of self-discovery can be emotionally taxing. It can generate a host of emotional reactions, ranging from denial to anger to hopelessness. Therefore, it is important to engage in self-care so that we are able to engage in effective self-reflection.

## ACTIVITY 8.1

Think about your identities. Next to each of the following, write down whether that aspect of your identity is considered a "norm" and part of a group that historically has been privileged (e.g., White, cisgender, affluent, male, nondisabled).

Race:

Gender:

Gender Identity:

Social Class:

Ethnicity:

Religion:

Nationality:

Language:

Of those you identified as being part of the dominant or "norm" group, think of a time you had negative reactions toward another who was different. What were your feelings? What was going on in your mind?

## Impairment

In Chapter 4, Professional Competence, we discussed our responsibility to acknowledge and respond appropriately if our personal functioning affects our work. In Chapter 7, Confronting Colleagues and Other Sticky Situations, we discussed how to respond if we notice unhealthy or unethical behavior in a colleague. But, what do we do when we notice, or someone tells us, that we are not functioning well? Proper self-care and self-awareness allow us to be open to acknowledging any impairment or limitations we may have. Without these, we may be more likely to deny or rationalize our behaviors or limitations.

There are a variety of responses to stress which can impact counselors' psychological functioning and work performance. However, it is important to differentiate psychological experiences that lead to some form of impairment from actual improper behavior. Wise et al. (2012) described "impairment" as "an objective change in the psychologist's professional functioning that may result in ineffective services or cause harm to those with whom we work" (p. 487). Examples of impairment included lateness with appointments or paperwork. Improper behavior, in contrast, constitutes a crossing of an ethical boundary and potential ethical misconduct. As discussed in Chapter 4, some of these improper behaviors include, for example, sexual contact with clients.

# SELF-ASSESSMENT: CURRENT BELIEFS AND EXPECTATIONS

## Instructions

If you were to take an essay test, how well would you be able to answer the following questions critically and thoroughly? Give yourself a letter grade A to F. Be honest; There are no right or wrong answers when learning where you stand.

## Beliefs Regarding Self-Care

- Role of the Counselor
  - What do you think is the role of a counselor in maintaining self-care? You may think of what your role does and does not consist of, as well as what you believe your responsibilities are.
  - What is the responsibility of the counselor regarding personal health and well-being?
  - What is the responsibility of a counselor in maintaining a workload that supports a healthy lifestyle?

- Function of Prioritizing Self-Care
    - What may be some benefits of modifying a workload or schedule?
    - In what ways are you competent and confident in your ability to recognize your personal and professional needs?
    - What personal factors may impede your ability to accurately identify issues and/or respond to them?
    - Think of cultural variables or situational variables that may impact your ability to effectively address your personal and professional needs.

## Expectations

- Successes in Treatment
    - What do you think is the role of self-care in the success of treatment?
    - What beliefs do you hold regarding "good counselors" and their ability to maintain self-care?
    - What are your current definitions of failure with regard to therapy, and what is your expectation of how effective you "should" be?
- Situations That May Be Challenging
    - In general, which types of situations or environments would create challenges for maintaining your self-care as a therapist?
- Situations That May Create Ethical Dilemmas
    - What are two situations that would *likely* create an ethical dilemma for you when dealing with issues related to self-care?
    - For you personally, what past experiences with burnout or self-care would likely impact your thinking and behavior?

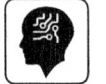

- Methods for Maintaining Self-Care
    - What do you actually do to maintain self-care? Think of immediate and ongoing actions as well as inner processes.

# ETHICAL STANDARDS SURROUNDING SELF-CARE

Both the American Psychological Association ([APA], 2017) and the American Counseling Association ([ACA], 2014) mention the management of or response to personal conflicts. However, terms such as *personal problems* or *self-care* are not specifically defined in either code of ethics. Rather, codes rely on the counselor's judgment of what would appropriately constitute a personal problem, as well as what would be appropriate self-care methods. Given the lack of specific direction, it is important to understand what is explicitly stated in the codes, and then follow up with additional education and training regarding these concepts.

References to the necessity of self-care can be found throughout each ethics code.

## APA's Ethical Principles of Psychologists and Code of Conduct

*Principle A: Beneficence and Nonmaleficence: Psychologists strive to benefit those with whom they work and take care to do no harm. In their professional actions, psychologists seek to safeguard the welfare and rights of those with whom they interact professionally and other affected persons, and the welfare of animal subjects of research. When conflicts occur among psychologists' obligations or concerns, they attempt to resolve these conflicts in a responsible fashion that avoids or minimizes harm. Because psychologists' scientific and professional judgments and actions may affect the lives of others, they are alert to and guard against personal, financial, social, organizational, or political factors that might lead to misuse of their influence. Psychologists strive to be aware of the possible effect of their own physical and mental health on their ability to help those with whom they work. (APA, 2017, p. 3)*

*APA Code 2.06, Personal Problems and Conflicts: (a) Psychologists refrain from initiating an activity when they know or should know that there is a substantial likelihood that their personal problems will prevent them from performing their work-related activities in a competent manner. (b) When psychologists become aware of personal problems that may interfere with their performing work-related duties adequately, they take appropriate measures, such as obtaining professional consultation or assistance, and determine whether they should limit, suspend, or terminate their work-related duties. (APA, 2017, p. 5)*

## ACA's Code of Ethics

ACA Code of Ethics, Section C: Professional Responsibility, includes the statement "counselors engage in self-care activities to maintain and promote their emotional, physical, mental, and spiritual well-being to best meet their professional responsibilities" (ACA, 2014, p. 8).

## DIFFERENCES AND OVERLAP

The preceding APA references, which fall under Standard 2, Competence, state the responsibility to notice impairment that has occurred as a result of personal problems as well as the responsibility to understand when to cease providing services as a result of these personal problems. Although APA mentions the need to address personal problems, the code does not address methods for maintaining personal and professional health. Notice that ACA's mention of self-care falls under the heading of professional responsibility and provides a direct mention of self-care and the need to maintain health in a variety of areas.

## Self-Care and Professional Behavior

The connection between self-care and ethical behavior lies in a counselor's ability to remain self-aware and to maintain effective judgment. A method for increasing these abilities is through self-care practices. When we are not taking care of ourselves, we can become much more likely to seek to have our intrapsychic/emotional/personal needs met through our work. Examples of needs that may be inappropriately met through work include:

- A need to feel powerful or important
- A need to feel useful or effective
- A need for closeness, a connection, or intimacy
- A need for a distraction from a personal situation
- A need to feel capable or intelligent
- A need to feel appreciated or needed

If counselors were aware that their needs were being met through their work, the result might be feelings such as shame or anxiety. Such negative emotions could consequently prevent counselors from being aware of their motivations or behavior. For example, a counselor may be pulling back from her relationships at home. To fill this need, she may begin to attach inappropriately to one particular client, albeit without conscious awareness of doing so. As a trained professional, this counselor would know that this is not a healthy way of engaging. In order to manage the anxiety that she would likely experience if she acknowledged the motivations underlying her behavior, she might remain unaware or in denial of her behavior. She may rationalize her actions by determining that this particular client was in need, and that they have developed a unique but effective connection. In this instance, the counselor may struggle to remain objective regarding her behavior in order to avoid feelings of shame and anxiety. This is precisely why regular self-care practices that promote self-awareness are critical for providing ethical and effective counseling services.

As counselors providing therapy, it is important to consistently monitor ourselves in our personal and work lives and determine if it is time to begin or return to therapy or some other form of focused support. Depending on the theoretical orientation, there are a variety of methods for understanding how counselors respond to their work. For assistance with this, clinical supervision that involves a focus on our internal dynamics and their interaction with our work can be significantly helpful and supportive in the quest to manage our inner experience and its effect on our work. Counseling can result in some internal conflicts or disrupted schemas. For example, we may at times be faced with some of life's harsh realities which may challenge our current worldviews. Examining these in therapy or supervision will be useful for maintaining healthy functioning and the ability to remain self-reflective.

Along with what has been mentioned thus far, we have additional practical recommendations:

1. *Develop and maintain a network of peers who can be called on for consultation or for support.* In order to develop an effective network of peers for consultation, it is wise to choose peers whom you respect but who are not close friends. Although you may have developed friendships with colleagues, keeping a separate group that can become closely acquainted with your work but remain objective is important.

2. *Identify another professional within your workplace who can serve as your self-care accountability partner.* Work with your colleague so that you may assist one another with maintaining healthy work habits. Specifically, discuss experiences with success and perceived failure, as well as beliefs regarding best practices and realistic expectations for outcomes. Work together not only to provide support, but to regularly challenge your beliefs and expectations in order to maintain a realistic and healthy personal worldview.

3. *Put thought and effort into designing a healthy work schedule* that will not put you at regular risk of burnout. Consider your work environment, amount of support, amount and intensity of your work responsibilities, and your personal situation. If you are not currently working as a counselor, imagine what the healthiest routine might be. If you are already working, think about what you need more or less of to maintain your health as well as your excellence in providing therapeutic services.

4. *Join a professional organization* that offers workshops and educational seminars for remaining up to date with local and national ethical standards, as well as opportunities for learning new methods for maintaining self-care. Professional organizations can provide a sense of community and of support, while providing up-to-date information and strategies for providing the best care for your clients.

## Dilemma: Recognizing When Our Personal Functioning or Reactions to Our Work May Be Impacting Our Effectiveness

A lack of self-care will negatively impact the quality of mental health services that a counselor provides. Stress and anxiety impact our ability to be perceptive and responsive to others.

## ACTIVITY 8.2

Explore the messages you have received regarding "being a psychologist" or "being a counselor." You have received many messages from media, colleagues, supervisors, and instructors. Identify as many as you can and write them down. For example, a common message we receive is "good psychologists know how to let things go, they don't take things personally at work." Another is "good counselors help most of their clients to feel and get better." Once you have identified the messages you have received, think about what they mean for you and your own expectations.

## VIGNETTES FOR DISCUSSION

### Instructions

In previous chapters we reviewed vignettes to practice identifying which ethical standards applied and how to proceed regarding a colleague or a client. Here, we review vignettes describing potential personal reactions that a counselor may have to his or her work. While reviewing these vignettes, you may choose to imagine that you are reading about yourself, or you may allow yourself to image how you would respond if this were a colleague or friend.

When reading the following short vignettes, remember to monitor your reactions, keeping track of any that include shaming the counselor for "bad" behavior or for being a "bad counselor." Focus on internal and external factors that may be impacting the counselors' behavior. Now is the time to notice if there are any patterns in your reactions, or the substance of your reactions, and to discuss these in supervision and consultation. This is valuable information for your reflection on what some of your personal biases and blind spots may be (see the Appendix, Typical Cognitive and Emotional Reactions, at the end of this book).

### Vignette 1

*Javier has been working with adolescents in a group home, providing individual and group counseling for the past 9 months. He began as an intern, but 2 months ago received his master's in counseling and is now a regular employee. He initially enjoyed working with adolescents; he learned to rely on supervision and other staff for support when he was feeling unsure or frustrated regarding his performance or effectiveness. Lately, however, he has been receiving less supervision, as he is expected to function more independently. His individual and group caseload has also doubled. Javier finds himself tired at work and looking forward to the end of the day, although once he is home he often finds himself thinking of work. He feels some pressure to be helpful and a "good counselor," but feels generally ineffective due to rejection that he experiences from some of the adolescents on his caseload.*

*(continued)*

## VIGNETTES FOR DISCUSSION (continued)

### Resolving the Ethical Dilemma

1. What information is relevant to understanding Javier's experience?
2. What additional information would you like to know to be able to best understand his experience?
3. What steps could Javier take to improve his experience at work and at home?
4. What steps could Javier take to improve his performance at work?
5. Which ethical codes may apply?
6. Would you determine Javier to be impaired in any way? If so, what conditions could have resulted in his impairment?

### Vignette 2

*Sheila has been working in a community mental health setting where she provides trauma-focused therapy for adolescents and adults. She began to work for this organization after she received additional training in trauma-focused work. Her employer was happy to have her, given the needs of the client population. Sheila quickly received many referrals from other counselors, increasing her caseload to 30 clients. She was initially hesitant, given her training and understanding that this type of work could be challenging. However, her employer offered her support and agreed to reduce her caseload if it became overwhelming. Sheila began to provide treatment and asked for support when she needed it. One year later, she began to call out of work regularly and was late with paperwork. She acknowledged that she felt stressed, but generally relied on relaxing on the weekend for relief. However, while at home Sheila began to feel a lack of connection with her partner and was generally dissatisfied. She also began to feel hopeless and caught herself ruminating about the types of trauma that she was hearing about at work. Sheila began to become avoidant of some social activities in an attempt to relax, but did not experience any relief.*

### Resolving the Ethical Dilemma

1. What information is relevant to understanding Sheila's experience?
2. What additional information would you like to know to be able to better understand her experience?
3. What steps could Sheila take to improve her experience at work and at home?
4. What steps could Sheila take to improve her performance at work?

*(continued)*

## VIGNETTES FOR DISCUSSION (continued)

5. Which ethical codes may apply?
6. Would you determine Sheila to be impaired in any way? If so, what conditions could have resulted in her impairment?

### Vignette 3

*Julia is working at an inpatient substance abuse center. She recently earned her doctoral degree and is working with clients who also experience some form of mental illness. Julia has a specific interest in substance abuse treatment. Before earning her doctoral degree, she was credentialed as a substance abuse counselor and worked in other treatment settings. Although Julia is not a supervisor, she holds a significant amount of responsibility. She is the only licensed doctoral-level counselor and so she is assigned all clients who have been diagnosed with a comorbid mental illness. Julia often struggles to manage her caseload while tasked with preparing for groups and other responsibilities. Recently, a client who had spent 6 months at the center was released. Julia had worked closely with him and felt invested in his progress and recovery. Julia felt sad to see him go as she had enjoyed her sessions with him more than other clients. Recently, while facilitating a group or sitting with other clients, Julia found herself thinking of this client. While at home, Julia also caught herself wishing that she could see this client again, as she was curious about his progress following his release. Also while at home, Julia had been feeling increasingly irritable and negative toward her partner as well as others in general. Her mother spoke with Julia regarding her concerns that Julia was "not herself."*

### Resolving the Ethical Dilemma

1. What information is relevant to understanding Julia's experience?
2. What additional information would you like to know to be able to better understand her experience?
3. What steps could Julia take to improve her experience at work and at home?
4. What steps could Julia take to improve her performance at work?
5. Which ethical codes may apply?
6. Would you determine Julia to be impaired in any way? If so, what conditions could have resulted in her impairment?

### Vignette 4

*Charles is a licensed psychologist who has been practicing for the past 15 years. He works in private practice along with two colleagues who share his office space. He sees a variety of clients, ranging from adolescents to adults who are experiencing a*

*(continued)*

> **VIGNETTES FOR DISCUSSION** (continued)
>
> range of symptoms and conditions. Charles often fills his schedule, as this represents his only income. He finds himself wishing that he could take time off but continues to schedule a full caseload of patients; this leaves him feeling overwhelmed and generally worn out. The last client that Charles sees each week is a 59-year-old man who has chronic obstructive pulmonary disease (COPD). This client struggles to breathe and is also struggling with issues relating to his illness and the end of his life. Recently, Charles caught himself listening to his own breathing, and feeling shortness of breath at times. Charles has also noticed that he has been ruminating about his client, often wishing that he could be more helpful or fantasizing that his client would be well again.
>
> **Resolving the Ethical Dilemma**
>
> 1. What information is relevant to understanding Charles's experience?
> 2. What additional information would you like to know to be able to better understand his experience?
> 3. What steps could Charles take to improve his experience at work and at home?
> 4. What steps could Charles take to improve his performance at work?
> 5. Which ethical codes may apply?
> 6. Would you determine Charles to be impaired in any way? If so, what conditions could have resulted in his impairment?

# CHAPTER DISCUSSION QUESTIONS

1. What are ways to differentiate between burnout, compassion fatigue, and vicarious trauma? What would be appropriate ways to respond to each condition?
2. What steps would you follow to engage in a self-care routine that would encompass all aspects of the model discussed in this chapter? Which aspects of this model would be difficult to address?
3. How can you create an interpersonal environment in which your colleagues or others close to you would be able to provide you with feedback regarding your personal and professional functioning?
4. For any of the vignettes noted in this chapter, assign sex, gender, sexual orientation, culture, socioeconomic standing, nation of origin, immigrant status, refugee status, primary language spoken, disability, or others. Would any of these variables impact your perception of the statements or actions within this vignette? If so, how? If not, what leads you to believe that none of these variables would impact your thinking or reactions? This information regarding your beliefs and reactions would be useful to discuss going forward in supervision.

# CONCLUSION

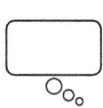

The ability to engage in ethical decision making and ethical behavior relies on two main skills. The first skill involves knowledge of the ethics codes and intellectual methods for decision making that are in line with the ethics codes. This includes the ability to properly navigate the decision-making tree as well as a strong understanding of what is required with regard to workplace rules and ethical standards. The second skill involves personal aspects of the counselor, such as your ability to effectively perceive and respond to ethical dilemmas based on your capacity for self-awareness and self-care. Both skills must be present. An intellectual understanding of the code, by itself, may not be sufficient, because a counselor can easily misperceive a situation based on internal variables such as motivations and schemas, as well as external variables that have impacted the counselor's internal experience, such as workplace norms or stressors. Self-care, described as a multicomponent process in this chapter, is essential for managing internal and external variables, and thus necessary for effective decision making when confronted with ethical dilemmas.

## PERSONAL INVENTORY: QUESTIONS FOR FURTHER EXPLORATION

### PROFESSIONAL EXPERIENCES

1. Have you had an experience in the past in which your boss, manager, or professional superior seemed to be impaired in some way, or lacking an appropriate amount of self-care? What was your reaction and response to this?

2. Have you had an experience at work or school in which you noticed policies or procedures that seemed to be in conflict with your ability to maintain self-care? What was your reaction and how did you respond?

### PERSONAL EXPERIENCES

1. Can you recall messages that you have received throughout your life regarding the need to engage in self-care? Reflect on messages you have received through your family of origin, your culture, and your training.

2. Do you remember a time in the past when you experienced a negative personal reaction to your work? Reflect on the variables of your work as well as your personal response.

## FURTHER LEARNING AND SUGGESTED READINGS

Goodman, G. (2005). "I feel stupid and contagious": Countertransference reactions of fledgling clinicians to patients who have negative therapeutic reactions. *American Journal of Psychotherapy, 59*, 149–168.

Pipher, M. (2003). *Letters to a young therapist: Stories of hope and healing*. New York, NY: Basic Books.

Warren, J., & Douglas, K. (2012). Falling from grace: Understanding an ethical sanctioning experience. *Counseling and Values, 57*, 131–146.

# REFERENCES

American Counseling Association. (2014). *2014 ACA code of ethics*. Retrieved from https://www.counseling.org/resources/aca-code-of-ethics.pdf

American Psychological Association. (2017). *Ethical principles of psychologists and code of conduct* (2002, amended June 1, 2010 and January 1, 2017). Retrieved from http://www.apa.org/ethics/code/index.aspx

Bamonti, P., Keelan, C., Larson, N., Mentrikoski, J., Randall, C., Sly, S., . . . McNeil, D. (2014). Promoting ethical behavior by cultivating a culture of self-care during graduate training: A call to action. *Training and Education in Professional Psychology, 8*, 253–260. doi:10.1037/tep0000056

Bianchi, R., & Schonfeld, S. (2015). Burnout is associated with a depressive cognitive style. *Personality and Individual Differences, 100*, 1–5. doi:10.1016/j.paid.2016.01.008

Brooks, S., Dunn, R., Amlôt, R., Greenberg, R., & Rubin, J. (2016). Social and occupational factors associated with psychological distress and disorder among disaster responders: A systematic review. *BMC Psychology, 4*, 1–13. doi:10.1186/s40359-016-0120-9

Burkholder, D., & Burkholder, J. (2014). Reasons for ethical misconduct of counseling students: What do faculty think? *Journal of Counselor Preparation and Supervision, 6*(2). doi:10.7729/52.1063

Colman, D., Echon, R., Lemay, M., McDonald, J., Smith, K., Spencer, J., & Swift, J. (2016). The efficacy of self-care for graduate students in professional psychology: A meta-analysis. *Training and Education in Professional Psychology, 10*, 188–197. doi:10.1037/tep0000130

Corey, G. (2013). *Theory and practice of counseling and psychotherapy* (9th ed.). Belmont, CA: Cengage.

Datillo, F. (2015). The self-care of psychologists and mental health professionals: A review and practitioner guide. *Australian Psychologist, 50*, 393–399. doi:10.1111/ap.12157

Gerber, M., Lang, C., Feldmeth, A., Elliot, C., Brand, S., Holsboer-Trachsler, E., & Pühse, U. (2015). Burnout and mental health in Swiss vocational students: The moderating role of physical activity. *Journal of Research on Adolescence, 25*(1), 63–74. doi:10.1111/jora.12097

Harrison, R., & Westwood, R. (2009). Preventing vicarious traumatization of mental health therapists: Identifying protective factors. *Psychotherapy Theory, Research, Practice, Training, 46*, 203–219. doi:10.1037/a0016081

Huggard, P. (2003). Compassion fatigue: How much can I give? *Medical Education, 37*, 163–164.

Johnson, H., Worthington, R., Gredecki, N., & Wilks-Riley, F. (2016). The relationship between trust in work colleagues, impact of boundary violations and burnout among staff within a forensic psychiatric service. *Journal of Forensic Practice, 18*, 64–75.

Joinson, C. (1992). Coping with compassion fatigue. *Nursing, 22*, 116–120.

Lee, J., Wallace, S., Puig, A., Choi, B., Nam, S., & Lee, S. (2010). Factor structure of the counselor burnout inventory in a sample of sex offender and sexual abuse therapists. *Measurements and Evaluation in Counseling and Development, 43*, 16–30. doi:10.1177/0748175610362251

Matula, B. (2013). Burnout/stress management: How to reduce burnout and stress in the workplace. *Journal of Healthcare Protection Management, 29*(1), 92–95.

Mazzula, S. L., & Nadal, L. (2015). Racial microaggressions, whiteness and feminist therapy. *Women and Therapy, 38*(3–4), 308–326.

Nadal, K. L. (2013). *That's so gay! Microaggressions and the lesbian, gay, bisexual, and transgender community.* Washington, DC: American Psychological Association.

Najjar, N., Davis, L., Beck-Coon, K., & Doebbeling, C. (2009). Compassion fatigue: A review of the research to date and relevance to cancer-care providers. *Journal of Health Psychology, 14*, 267–277.

Pearlman, L., & Mac Ian, P. (1995). Vicarious traumatization: An empirical study of the effects of trauma work on trauma therapists. *Professional Psychology: Research and Practice, 26*, 558–565.

Shim, R. S., Compton, M. T., Rust, G., Druss, B. G., & Kaslow, N. J. (2009). Race-ethnicity as a predictor of attitudes toward mental health treatment seeking. *Psychiatric Services, 60*(10), 1336–1341.

Smith, L., & Redington, R. M. (2010). Lessons from the experiences of White antiracist activists. *Professional Psychology: Research and Practice, 41*, 541–549.

Sweeney, J., & Creaner, M. (2014). What's not being said? Recollections of nondisclosure in clinical supervision while in training. *British Journal of Guidance & Counselling, 42*(2), 211–224. doi:10.1080/03069885.2013.872223

Testa, D., & Sangganjanavanich, V. (2015). Contribution of mindfulness and emotional intelligence to burnout among counseling interns. *Counselor Education & Supervision, 55*, 95–108. doi:10.1002/ceas.12035

Thompson, V. L. S., Bazile, A., & Akbar, M. (2004). African-Americans' perceptions of psychotherapy and psychotherapists. *Professional Psychology: Research and Practice, 35*(1), 19–26.

Toker, S., & Biron, M. (2012). Job burnout and depression: Unraveling their temporal relationship and considering the role of physical activity. *Journal of Applied Psychology, 97*, 699–710. doi:10.1037/a0026914

Turner, J., Edwards, L., Eicken, I., Yokoyama, K., Castro, J., Ncog-Thuy Tran, A., & Haggins, K. (2005). Intern self-care: An exploratory study into strategy use and effectiveness. *Professional Psychology: Research and Practice, 36,* 674–680. doi:10.1037/0735-7028.36.6.674

Wei, X., Wang, R., & MacDonald, E. (2015). Exploring the relations between student cynicism and student burnout. *Psychological Reports: Employment Psychology & Marketing, 117,* 103–115. doi:10.2466/14.11.PR0.117c14z6

Wise, E., Hersh, M., & Gibson, C. (2012). Ethics, self-care and well-being for psychologists: Reenvisioning the stress-distress continuum. *Professional Psychology: Research and Practice, 43,* 487–494. doi:10.1037/a0029446

# CHAPTER 9

# COUNSELORS AND BEYOND

Our intention in creating this book was to provide a comprehensive and effective method for learning and applying ethical codes and standards. We believe that ethical behavior is contingent upon three variables: knowledge of the codes and how they are applied, internal factors or those specific to the counselor, and external factors such as environmental conditions.

This book presented a series of common ethical dilemmas and provided a roadmap for how to identify and apply the appropriate ethical standards, while considering the necessary contextual variables (internal and external factors). Going forward, it is our hope that counselors develop this method for analyzing their behavior in response to their work.

An underlying intention for this book was to create an environment in which counselors remain open to embracing their individuality and humanness—an environment in which counselors are trained to avoid shaming themselves and others, and rather engage in a compassionate look at their own and others' functioning. We believe that counselors must acknowledge their vulnerability to engaging in unethical behavior, given the circumstances. Phillip Zimbardo, who provided us with a classic example of how power and situational variables drastically impact behavior through his Stanford Prison Study, has since stated:

*As my own experiment revealed, and as a great deal of social-psychological research before and since has confirmed, we humans exaggerate the extent to which our actions are voluntary and rationally chosen—or, put differently, we all understate the power of the situation. (Zimbardo, 2007, p. B6)*

With this knowledge in mind, it is a counselor's responsibility to recognize factors that may impede his or her ability to behave in an ethical manner and take steps to create a situation that results in sound judgment. Our goal was to assist in this process.

In this final chapter, we provide recommendations regarding the development and maintenance of ethical practices, as well as summary messages for trainees and early career counselors, supervisors, and training programs. Our recommendations are grounded in our clinical experiences, including our theoretical orientations, as well as our training, research, and teaching approach. In providing recommendations, we readily acknowledge that some are not new, and have been discussed by previous scholars and researchers. We bridge the fields of mental health counseling, counseling psychology, and clinical psychology, as well as other fields of study including multicultural, health, and social psychology. Our recommendations are person-centered, with attention to the multiple variables that impact functioning, including the environment and group memberships. We also review ethical codes and standards of both the American Psychological Association (APA) and the American Counseling Association (ACA) as they relate to self-care and requirements regarding responding to ethical complaints.

# TAKE-HOME DISCUSSION QUESTIONS

## Academic and Informational

1. Reflecting on the ethical standards and dilemmas discussed throughout the book, what questions remain regarding ethics and counseling?
2. Regarding your specific educational or training program, which areas could be expanded or improved in order to provide proper preparation for managing some of the ethical dilemmas discussed?
3. Regarding the specific set of ethical standards that govern your professional roles (e.g., APA or ACA), which areas could be expanded or improved in order to provide proper preparation for managing some of the ethical dilemmas discussed?
4. Identify changes in your knowledge or opinions that have occurred during your reading of this book. Looking back, were there misconceptions that have now been corrected given this information regarding ethical standards and dilemmas?

## Self-Reflective

1. What are specific areas that were previously anxiety provoking that are now less so given your increase in knowledge and practice with thinking them through?
2. Reflect on the vignettes that were presented throughout this book. Is there one that has stuck with you or was particularly memorable? Why do you believe this was?
3. Given your understanding of how ethical violations can occur, have you begun to revise your understanding of what a "good counselor" is? Does your understanding of ethical behavior include contextual reasons for which counselors engage in inappropriate behavior?
4. This may be hard to do, but give it a try. Can you imagine contextual factors that would increase your likelihood of acting in an inappropriate manner? Think of environmental factors as well as personal factors. Which combination of factors might put you at risk?

## TAKE-HOME PLANS

- Identify partners, whether colleagues or classmates, who will be able to serve as "self-care accountability partners" or "ethics accountability partners" at this time or moving forward throughout your respective careers.
  - Together, identify qualities of an effective accountability partner, as well as ways that each could serve as a helpful source of support.
  - Make plans to create opportunities for regular contact in order to openly discuss concerns that arise in reaction to counseling work.
- Research and identify a professional organization that appears to be offering an interesting ethics-related workshop within the next 6 months. Choose one that is financially and practically possible for you to attend and make plans to do so. If possible, bring a colleague, classmate, or peer.
- Create a list of self-care questions that you will refer to and can ask yourself on a regular basis. This may include questions such as "Am I feeling energized?" or "Am I feeling increasingly frustrated at work?" At the bottom of the list, identify a person you can call to discuss this, as well as three immediate steps that you could take to begin to engage in self-care practices. These may include "seek professional consultation" or "increase my participation in mindfulness activities."

## MESSAGES FROM THE AUTHORS

### A Message to Trainees and Early Career Counselors

You are in a developmental period of your professional life that will end with you moving on to a fulfilling and exciting career. You have an opportunity to grow and challenge your beliefs in response to your training and work experiences. For you and your clients' benefit, remain open, flexible, and compassionate with yourself.

We described throughout this book the many ways in which counseling work can be confusing and challenging. Yet, with these skills and support, you will be able to navigate these experiences while gaining a truer understanding of yourself and others. Your understanding of your work today will likely change throughout your career; your responsibility is to ensure that you return to a place of understanding and openness as opposed to cynicism and rigidity.

Take note of some of the recommendations provided here regarding your continued development and methods for support. One of the benefits of this career is that it is full of other professionals who are available to connect with and learn from. Your goal will be to create circumstances that will best allow you to remain aware of contextual factors that may impact your judgment and functioning, and to assist your colleagues with doing the same.

# A Message to Supervisors and Educators

Counselors-in-training are in the midst of a unique developmental stage. They are still learning the fundamentals of theory and practice and having their initial experiences with practicums and internships. Early career counselors are still developing their professional identity, navigating conflicts between ethical guidelines and standards of practice and crystallizing their theoretical orientations and expertise. These initial experiences will have a significant impact on their approach to this work, as they will serve as a primary point of reference throughout their careers.

It is our responsibility as educators and supervisors to be mindful of the counselor's newly developing schemas and understandings of professional roles, and to guide each person to develop positive and realistic views of themselves and others with whom they will work. We should inform students and trainees to expect that their understandings of the world will be challenged by this work, and that their goal is to renegotiate their understandings in a way that rejects cynicism.

As educators and supervisors, we must be mindful of our students' training and professional identity. In the past, there were distinct differences in the functions of the specialty fields of mental health, counseling psychology, and clinical psychology. Depending on the setting, this is not always the case. Licensed Professional Counselors, Counseling Psychologists, and Clinical Psychologists are entering similar spaces and negotiating similar ethical dilemmas. While the ethical codes and standards of the APA and of the ACA share similarities in how they inform professional behavior, they vary by amount of detail and guidance provided; what is directly mentioned versus assumed; and, in some instances, the focus of their principles. Therefore, it is our responsibility to keep abreast of developing counselors' professional identities and be prepared to address ethical dilemmas in ways that are consistent with their guiding standards.

It is also our responsibility as educators and supervisors to provide direction for how to effectively engage in the educational and supervisory experience, as some students may not be open to or understand the process. We should be mindful of the motivations for students and trainees to avoid disclosing what they perceive to be negative reactions or behaviors. We should be offering regular explanations of the utility of supervisory relationships, as well as suggestions for ways to acknowledge the wish to avoid disclosing with a supervisor, yet choosing to do so. Of course, the supervisory relationship must be experienced as safe in order for this to happen.

As supervisors and educators, we must also be attentive to the power dynamics inherent in our relationships with trainees, students, and early-career counselors, and create circumstances that will best allow us to remain aware of contextual factors that may impact our judgment and functioning.

# EDUCATION, TRAINING, AND SUPERVISION

## Review of Ethical Standards

### APA Ethical Principles of Psychologists and Code of Conduct

Whereas the American Psychological Association (2017) provides Standard 7, Education and Training, there are no codes that directly address teaching ethics. There are also no specific requirements of education outside of the need to provide "appropriate knowledge and proper experiences, and to meet the requirements for licensure, certification or other goals for which claims are made by the program" (APA, 2017, Code 7.01). This code speaks to those who are "responsible for education and training programs," specifically. In this case, APA offers several other codes, including requirements on adequate description of program content, goals, and objectives (Code 7.02, Descriptions of Education and Training Programs).

APA does, however, include guidelines around disclosure of personal information in program-related activities, in Code 7.04, Student Disclosure of Personal Information:

> *Psychologists do not require students or supervisees to disclose personal information in course- or program-related activities, either orally or in writing, regarding sexual history, history of abuse and neglect, psychological treatment, and relationships with parents, peers, and spouses or significant others except if (1) the program or training facility has clearly identified this requirement in its admissions and program materials or (2) the information is necessary to evaluate or obtain assistance for students whose personal problems could reasonably be judged to be preventing them from performing their training- or professionally related activities in a competent manner or posing a threat to the students or others. (APA, 2017, p. 10)*

As noted throughout the book, there may be additional codes and standards one must consult. For example, APA explicitly directs counselors engaged in teaching or training to review standards around boundaries of competence (Standard 2.03, Maintaining Competence; see Chapter 3).

### ACA Code of Ethics

The ACA Code of Ethics (ACA, 2014) provides direction regarding educational programs, as does APA. However, the ACA code provides additional guidelines on specific topics, including teaching of ethics (Code F.7.e, Teaching Ethics) and diversity (Code F.7.c, Infusing Multicultural Issues/Diversity).

The ACA ethics code includes statements regarding the role of educators in addressing concerns regarding their students' personal functioning, and also on counselors' self-growth requirements.

> *Code F.8.d., Addressing Personal: Concerns: Counselor educators may require students to address any personal concerns that have the potential to affect professional competency. (ACA, 2014, p. 14)*

*Code F.8.c., Self-Growth Experiences*: Self-growth is an expected component of counselor education. Counselor educators are mindful of ethical principles when they require students to engage in self-growth experiences. Counselor educators and supervisors inform students that they have a right to decide what information will be shared or withheld in class. (ACA, 2014, p. 14)

# Recommendations

## Recommendations for Educators

- While providing instruction regarding professional ethics, deter students from using language such as "a bad psychologist" or "a bad counselor," as well as a "good" psychologist or counselor. These types of rigid categories may negatively impact their understanding of themselves. If, at some point in their career, they engage in inappropriate behavior, they may remain in denial or rationalize their behavior due to their belief that they are "good" and incapable of "bad" behavior. We must impart the message early on that any person is capable of uncharacteristic behavior given certain circumstances.

- Reject a student's use of terms such as *crazy* when describing other professionals' unethical behavior. This provides the opportunity to practice nonshaming or nuanced thought around behavior as opposed to restricted or character-blaming thought. This will also allow students to acknowledge their own vulnerabilities and risk for engaging in similar unethical actions. Furthermore, it will enhance the development of nuanced thinking regarding clients' behavior.

- When providing case examples of ethical dilemmas, encourage students to identify the most anxiety-provoking aspect of the scenario. This will provide information regarding their understanding of their role as a counselor as well as fears they may have regarding counseling and relationships.

- When providing case examples of ethical dilemmas, encourage students to identify as many contextual factors as possible that may be impacting the counselor and client's points of view or experiences.

## Recommendations for Supervisors

- Monitor supervisees' cognitive, emotional, and behavioral response to ambiguity with regard to ethical dilemmas, and deter any attempts to quickly categorize actions based on a need to quickly resolve a dilemma. Teach your method for tolerating ambiguity as well as discomfort with regard to ethical dilemmas.

- Encourage supervisees to regularly report their self-care methods as well as any needs to modify these methods based on their reaction to their work.
- Although your supervisees may not be in a position to modify their workload, encourage them to identify how their workload may be impacting their performance or functioning. Offer your methods for creating a workload and work environment that allows for maintenance of self-care and ethical practice.
- Understand supervisees' professional identity and be prepared to address ethical dilemmas in ways that are consistent with their guiding standards and the profession's philosophical underpinnings.
- Offer open descriptions of your struggles with managing ethics, specifically around anxiety-producing areas such as boundaries or managing high workloads.
- Be flexible and compassionate with yourself to remain present in understanding when individual, cultural, or environmental factors impact how you engage supervisees and how you understand their experiences.
- Engage in self-care to continue providing sound supervision and ethical guidance.

## Recommendations for Training Programs

- Create an environment that is nonshaming around ethical dilemmas and professional behavior. Trainees will be less likely to fully acknowledge their behavior if they feel at risk for a strong negative emotional reaction from their educators or peers. For trainees, this is an opportunity to begin the practice of self-reflection in a nonthreatening environment that focuses on personal development and flexible problem solving.
- Create a learning competency that includes a trainee's effective methods for self-care and personal health practices. This may be done through a dedicated course, but should also be included as an aspect of any practicum or internship seminar classes.
- Facilitate opportunities for trainees to engage in dialogue around self-care practices as well as methods for effectively managing time and other components of the training experience.
- Encourage students to join national or state-level professional organizations so that they may remain abreast of changes regarding professional and ethical guidelines and regulations.
- Have readily available material on national, state, and institutional guidelines regarding ethical behavior, including

websites and contact information, in a centralized location that students can access.

# RESPONDING TO ETHICAL COMPLAINTS

## Review of Ethical Standards

### APA Ethical Principles of Psychologists and Code of Conduct

APA Code 1.06, Cooperating with Ethics Committees:

*Psychologists cooperate in ethics investigations, proceedings, and resulting requirements of the APA or any affiliated state psychological association to which they belong. In doing so, they address any confidentiality issues. Failure to cooperate is itself an ethics violation. However, making a request for deferment of adjudication of an ethics complaint pending the outcome of litigation does not alone constitute noncooperation. (APA, 2017, p. 4)*

APA Code 1.07, Improper Complaints:

*Psychologists do not file or encourage the filing of ethics complaints that are made with reckless disregard for or willful ignorance of facts that would disprove the allegation. (APA, 2017, p. 5)*

APA Code 1.08, Unfair Discrimination Against Complainants and Respondents:

*Psychologists do not deny persons employment, advancement, admissions to academic or other programs, tenure, or promotion, based solely upon their having made or their being the subject of an ethics complaint. This does not preclude taking action based upon the outcome of such proceedings or considering other appropriate information. (APA, 2017, p. 5)*

### ACA Code of Ethics

ACA I.3., Cooperation With Ethics Committees:

*Counselors assist in the process of enforcing the ACA Code of Ethics. Counselors cooperate with investigations, proceedings, and requirements of the ACA Ethics Committee or ethics committees of other duly constituted associations or boards having jurisdiction over those charged with a violation. (ACA, 2014, p. 19)*

ACA I.2.e., Unwarranted Complaints:

*Counselors do not initiate, participate in, or encourage the filing of ethics complaints that are retaliatory in nature or are made with reckless disregard or willful ignorance of facts that would disprove the allegation. (ACA, 2014, p. 19)*

ACA I.2.f., Unfair Discrimination Against Complainants and Respondents:

*Counselors do not deny individuals employment, advancement, admission to academic or other programs, tenure, or promotion based solely on their having made or their being the subject of an ethics complaint. This does not preclude taking action based on the outcome of such proceedings or considering other appropriate information. (ACA, 2014, p. 19)*

## Differences and Overlap

Notice that both the APA and ACA codes state the requirement for cooperation with ethics committees, specify the prohibited act of submitting "improper" or "unwarranted complaints," and (with almost exactly matching language) prohibit unfair discrimination against a psychologist/counselor just for having had a complaint filed against them, not precluding actions taken based on the outcome of the complaint.

## Practical Steps in Responding to an Ethics Complaint

You must respond; but before you do, reach out for social and legal support.

1. Contact your malpractice insurance provider to inform them of the complaint. You may qualify for an attorney through your insurance, but either way the insurer must be informed.

2. Consult an attorney before responding to the letter that you received from the ethics board. Do not attempt to contact the client/entity regarding the ethics complaint, and only communicate with your lawyer regarding the details.

3. Seek support. This is the time to create a support network, including colleagues and those within your personal circle. It is also time to acknowledge that the situation will likely lead to a significant amount of stress; thus, increased attention to maintaining self-care is needed in order to maintain healthy functioning.

## Practical Recommendations for Ethical Practices

1. Receive training regarding clinical/counseling notes. You will likely receive training at any practicum or internship sites where you work. However, every organization has different standards. You may wish to attend a webinar or other trainings focused on note taking in order to create therapy notes that are accurate, appropriate, and ethical.

2. There are ethical standards regarding record keeping (APA Standard 6: Record Keeping and Fees; ACA A.1.b., Records and Documentation). However, there may also be state or organizational guidelines that you will need to follow. Receive specific guidance and direction in this area to avoid any inappropriate records or disposals of records.

3. Keep records of all continuing education credits that you earned by attending workshops or trainings.

4. Keep notes and reminders for maintaining your professional license by paying dues, and always inform the licensing board if you change your address.
5. Regarding malpractice insurance, even if you are not required by your program to purchase malpractice insurance, it is wise to do so. As with other types of insurance, you may not see the need for it until the need arises. At that time, you will be grateful that you purchased insurance, as legal fees or lawsuits can be costly.

# RECOMMENDATIONS FOR FURTHER DEVELOPMENT

## Identifying Professional Support

- Each state's psychological or counseling association will have resources for responding to ethical dilemmas. You may need to be a member in order to access these resources, so it may be wise to investigate the fees associated with membership as well as groups that you could join within the organization aimed at providing practical support.
- Within APA and ACA, there are divisions for specialties or areas of interest. If you will be a member of either organization, it will be wise to also join a division where you will receive up-to-date research and recommendations for effective and ethical practices.
- Within your local community, there may be opportunities for privately established peer supervision or consultation groups. Often, these groups are ongoing and long term, which allows for more individualized and meaningful assistance with thinking through cases and ethical dilemmas. Although this would be a commitment, it would be an effective method for remaining attentive to any variables that are impacting your professional functioning.

## Recommendations for Continued Training

- Irrespective of your current area of interest, there will be opportunities for continued learning and training. These may be offered by state or private organizations. Make plans to immediately begin to regularly attend or participate in these experiences. There may be webinars or in-person workshops or seminars. Remaining connected to your interest will assist with preventing a sense of monotony or boredom with your work.
- Create a network of peers who share your professional interests and with whom you can share ideas and attend trainings.

- Continually reflect on your areas of competence as well as ways that you can increase or maintain your competence in these areas.

## Recommendations for Counselors and Social Responsibility

- Begin to identify ways in which you could contribute to the field through writing or verbally sharing your experiences at conferences or professional meetings. Your contribution to the field will not only be valuable to others, but will also promote your own pattern of continued learning and development.
- Find ways to share your knowledge with the public. If you go on to do research, find ways to de-jargonize the language so that the information can be shared directly with people outside of academia.
- Invest in an understanding of how politics affect the mental health of the country, as well as your individual work and the communities that you serve.
- Remember to mentor others once you have achieved some success. This should be a cooperative process that will only benefit the people we serve if we work closely together in support and through mentorship.

# CONCLUSION

In this chapter, we reviewed recommendations for teaching ethics within academic settings and for providing supervision. Maintaining ethical behavior is an ongoing and career-long process, so we also offered suggestions for ways to gain social and professional support regarding maintenance of ethical behavior. We also offered guidelines for responding to ethical complaints if they occur. As you move forward, remain open in your approach to reflecting on yourself, your actions, and your personal and professional needs, knowing that ethical situations will arise that will require new training, knowledge, or supervision that you will need in order to maintain ethical judgment and behavior. Your task is to continue with this learning and self-reflection throughout your career.

# RESOURCES

## Websites

American Board of Professional Psychology—www.abpp.org

American Counseling Association—www.counseling.org

American Counseling Association Foundation—http://acafoundation.org

American Mental Health Counselors Association—http://connections.amhca.org/home

American Psychological Association—www.apa.org

APA Practice Organization—www.apapracticecentral.org/ce/tools

Association for Counselor Education and Supervision—www.acesonline.net

Association for Multicultural Counseling and Development—www.multiculturalcounseling.org

Council for Accreditation of Counseling and Related Educational Programs (CACREP)—www.cacrep.org

Counselors for Social Justice—https://counseling-csj.org

National Board for Certified Counselors—http://nbcc.org

Professional Development Resources—www.pdresources.org

# REFERENCES

American Counseling Association. (2014). *2014 ACA code of ethics*. Alexandria, VA: Author.

American Psychological Association. (2017). *Ethical principles of psychologists and code of conduct* (2002, amended June 1, 2010 and January 1, 2017). Retrieved from http://www.apa.org/ethics/code/index.aspx

Zimbardo, P. G. (2007). Revisiting the Stanford prison experiment: A lesson in the power of situation. *Chronicle of Higher Education, 53*(30), B6.

# APPENDIX

## TYPICAL COGNITIVE AND EMOTIONAL REACTIONS

Our ability to properly identify and address our reactions to dilemmas is contingent upon our level of self-awareness, or ability to accurately label and experience our cognitive and emotional reactions. These lists are by no means comprehensive; rather, they are offered as a guide to begin to acknowledge your reactions, especially those that may be uncomfortable. Most importantly, remember that there are no "bad" reactions. Rather, it is our responsibility to be as honest as possible with our reactions so that we can manage them properly.

| COGNITIVE | EMOTIONAL |
|---|---|
| Clarity | Concerned |
| Unclear | Unconcerned |
| Openness | Attentive |
| Closed | Inattentive |
| Flexibility | Caring |
| Inflexible | Uncaring |
| Overloaded | Worried |
| Distracted | Relaxed |
| Stuck | Anxious |
| Curious | Fearful |
| Confident | Nervous |
| Unsure | Frustrated |
| Interested | Proud |
| Uninterested | Confident |
| Motivated | Unconfident |
| Avoidant | Angry |
| Black and white | Annoyed |

- Grey
- Nuanced
- Fixated
- Problem-focused
- Blame-focused
- Solution-focused
- Excited
- Compassionate
- Relieved
- Hopeful
- Hopeless
- Helpless
- Capable

# INDEX

accepting gifts, 39, 41–42
acculturation, 74, 82
advertising, 99, 107
American Counseling Association's (ACA) Code of Ethics
    confidentiality, 22
    culturally competent treatment, 79–80, 89–92
    ethical complaints, 176–177
    institutional resources, 7
    introduction to ethical standards, 3–4
    issue identification, 7
    national resources, 7
    professional boundaries, 41–44
    professional competence, 56–57, 61–62
    professional support, 178
    review of standards, 176–177
    rule of law, 5–6
    social media, 106–108, 110, 112–113, 116
    state resources, 7
    sticky situations, 125–127, 133–134, 136–137
    structure, 4
American Psychological Association's (APA) Code of Ethics
    colleagues' behavior, 126–130, 133–135
    confidentiality, 21–25, 27–29
    culturally competent treatment, 78–81
    education and training, 173
    ethical complaints, 176
    introduction to ethical standards, 3–4
    professional boundaries, 41–44
    professional competence, 55–59
    professional support, 178
    rule of law, 5–6
    self-awareness, 91–92
    self-care, 157–158
    social media, 99, 101, 105–109
    structure, 4

blind spots, 12, 45, 60, 85, 91–92, 107, 111, 131, 137, 147, 149, 161
boundary crossings, 35–36
boundary violations, 35–36
burnout, 28, 145, 148, 150, 152, 157, 160, 164, 166

case studies
    confidentiality, 31–33
    professional boundaries, 44–46
    professional competence, 62–64
    social media, 118
    sticky situations, 137–139
citizenship status, 74, 77, 149
client
    boundary violations with, 36
    confidentiality, 19–22
    contemporary issues, 87–89
    intercultural differences, 37–38
    personal stress, 60
    providing information, 50–53, 124
    psychological assessments, 72
    quality of life, 145
    sociopolitical factors, 74–79
    –therapist relationship, 3–6, 149, 151
    trauma experience, 153
    virtual space, 97–98, 100, 102–104, 116
    worldview impacts, 81–84
clinical psychology, 8, 169, 172
clinical supervision, 147, 159
compassion fatigue, 145, 152–153
competence
    cultural, 71–74, 78–80, 83, 91
    professional, 3, 49–66
confidentiality
    ACA Code of Ethics, 22
    APS's standard, 21–22
    beliefs regarding, 20–21

confidentiality *(cont.)*
   case study, 31–33
   definition, 19
   exceptions, 28–31
   expectations, 21
   need for discussion, 22–24
   third-party authorization, 24–28
consultation
   client's privacy, 22, 25, 27
   cultural competency, 58, 98
   necessary training and skill, 52
   professional boundaries, 35
   professional development, 150, 158
   self-care elements, 147
   self-disclosure, 42
   specific situation, 6, 61
   support system, 122
consultation groups, 150, 178
continuing education, 49, 62, 72, 83, 177
Council for Accreditation of Counseling & Related Educational Programs (CACREP), 6, 8
counseling psychology, 8, 169, 172
counselors
   colleagues' behavior, 124–125
   common lawsuits, 5
   confidentiality, dealing, 20–21
   cultural competence, 73–74
   duty to warn, 6
   professional boundaries, 39–40
   professional competence, 54–55
   self-care, 156–157
   social media management, 105–106
countertransference, 147
Credentialed Alcoholism and Substance Abuse Counselor (CASAC), 9
criminal justice system, 24, 26–27, 32
critical self-reflections
   cultural competence, 72
   self-awareness and, 14–15, 91–92, 154
   socially constructed privileges, 154
cultural norms
   informal resolution, 129
   professional boundaries, 36–39
   time preference, 87
   workplace and, 121
culture
   boundaries of competence, 58–59
   collectivism, 82
   confidentiality and privacy, 22
   online, 97
   Western, 88
   workplace, 10, 37, 121
   worldviews, 84

*Diagnostic and Statistical Manual of Mental Disorders (DSM-5)*, 71, 75–76
dialectical behavioral therapy, 50–51
digital natives, 102
disability, 77
discrimination, 76–77
doctoral-level students, 8–9, 101, 103
dual degrees, 8
dual relationships, 36

early career, 4, 102, 149, 169, 171–172
ethical dilemmas
   confidentiality, 22–24, 28–30, 115–116
   confronting colleagues, 127–130, 136–137
   gifts, accepting, 42–43
   inappropriate relationship, 43–44
   level of competence, counselors, 56–60
   maintaining professional competence, 62
   personal situation, 60–62
   self-disclosure, 41–42
   social media representation, 112–113
   sticky situation, 133–134, 136–137
   third-party authorization, 24–28
   virtual relationships, 109–110
ethical standards
   colleagues' behavior, 125–126
   confidentiality, 21–22
   culturally competent treatment, 78–80
   governing bodies, 3–4
   personal reactions to work, 160
   professional boundaries, 40–41
   professional competence, 55–56
   self-care, 157–158
   social media, 106–109

Facebook, 98–102, 106, 119
formal resolution, 127–128, 130

general understanding, 50–52
gray areas, 36, 41, 44

homosexuality, 76

inappropriate relationships, 39, 41, 43
informal resolution, 121, 125, 127–130
informed consent, 23–26, 28, 32, 89, 110, 113, 116, 136
internal dynamics, 36–37
invitations, 88–89

judgment, 11, 15, 97, 149–151, 153–154, 158–159, 169, 172, 179

knowledge, 9, 11, 49–50, 52, 62, 72, 82–83, 91, 101, 165

language, 23, 31, 46, 71–72, 75–76, 80, 102, 155
lesbian, gay, bisexual, transgender, and queer (LGBTQ), 58, 75–77

Masters in Psychology and Counseling Accreditation Council (MPCAC), 6, 8
master's-level students, 8–9
mental health programs, 8
multicultural competence, 12, 37, 50, 57, 72, 79

necessary training and skills, 50–53

organizational conflicts, 133–134

peer supervision, 178
personal problems, 11, 38, 61, 158
predoctoral students, 8–9
professional boundaries
    ACA Code of Ethics, 41
    accepting gifts, 42–43
    APA standards, 41
    beliefs, 39–40
    case study, 44–46
    crossing, 35
    cultural norms, 36–38
    expectations, 40
    inappropriate relationships, 43–44
    self-disclosure, 41–42
    slippery slope, 36
    violations, 35
    workplace norms, 38–39
professional competence
    ACA Code of Ethics, 55
    APA standards, 55
    areas of interest, 62
    assessment of ability, 56–60
    assigning trainees, 52–53
    beliefs, 54
    case study, 62–64
    definition, 49–50
    ethical standards, 55
    expectations, 54–55
    general understanding about clients, 50–51
    maintaining, 62
    necessary for training and skills, 50–52
    personal situations, 60–61
    self-assessment, 54–55

quality of life, 145

racism, 76–77
receiving gifts, 11, 42–44, 46
religion, 77–78
rumination, 61, 162

self-awareness
    ACA Code of Ethics, 79–80
    client–counselor therapeutic relationship, 12
    critical role, 28
    cultural competencies, 91–93
    development and practice, 13
    emotional reactions, 181
    ethical decision making, 15
    personal therapy, 149
    professional behavior, 159
    purpose of self-care, 153–154
    socially constructed privileges, 154
    vicarious traumatization, 153
self-care
    counselor's engagement, 146–147
    elements, 147–151
    need for, 146
    self-awareness and, 153–154
self-disclosure, 38–39, 41–42, 44, 46, 88, 102
sexual orientation disorder, 76
slippery slope, 36, 122
social identities, 14–15
social media
    ACA Code of Ethics, 108–109
    accuracy, information, 112–115
    APA standards, 107–108
    benefits, 100–101
    case study, 118
    confidentiality, 115–116
    counseling version, 98–99
    disadvantages, 101–105
    privacy settings, 99–100
    virtual relationships, 109–110
social support, 82, 147
specialty training, 14, 49, 57–58, 62, 172

supervision
  boundary crossings, 35, 37, 42, 88
  group, 128
  personal situation, 61
  professional competence, 49, 51–53, 62–63
  self-care, 147–150
  training and, 59, 129

therapy
  conversion, 76
  family, 82
  group, 58
  individual, 81–82, 87
  in-home, 88
time preference, 87
transgender and gender nonconforming, 75–77
treatment, sociopolitical realities
  acculturation, 74
  citizenship status, 74
  disability, 77
  discrimination, 76–77
  gender roles, 75
  language, 75
  lesbian, gay, bisexual, or queer individuals, 75–76
  racism, 76–77
  religion, 77–78
  social class, 77
  transgender and gender nonconforming, 75–76

undergraduate-level students, 9

vicarious trauma, 152–153

workplace norms, 36–38
  accepting gifts, 39, 41–43
  inappropriate relationships, 39, 41, 43
  self-disclosure, 38–39, 41–42, 44, 46
worldviews, 32, 71–72
  boundary crossings, 87–88
  cultural competency, 81–84
  schemas, 150
  self-care, 154, 160